POSTCARD CATS

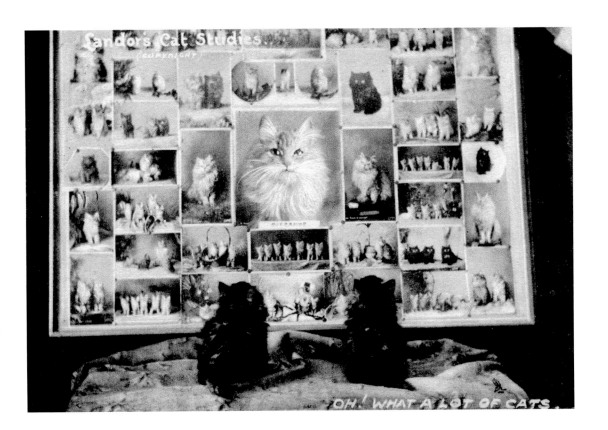

POSTCARD CATS

LIBBY HALL & TOM PHILLIPS

BLOOMSBURY

First published in Great Britain in 2005

Copyright © 2005 by Libby Hall and Tom Phillips

The moral right of the authors has been asserted

Bloomsbury Publishing Plc,
36 Soho Square, London W1D 3QY

A CIP catalogue record for this book is available from the British Library

ISBN 0 7475 8095 2
ISBN-13 9780747580959

10 9 8 7 6 5 4 3 2 1

Designed by William Webb
Printed and bound by L.E.G.O. S.p.A, Vicenza, Italy

All papers used by Bloomsbury Publishing are natural, recyclable products
made from wood grown in well-managed forests. The manufacturing processes
conform to the environmental regulations of the country of origin.

www.postcardcats.com

INTRODUCTION

Cats and human beings are old friends. We have long been familiar with the cats of the ancient Egyptians, drawn and sculpted 5,000 years ago, or intricately bound as mummies with ears made of linen and painted faces. However, it is only very recently that we have learned how far back in time the pedigree of the relationship actually extends. Archaeologists digging at a funerary site in Cyprus in 2004 chanced upon a grave in which the bones of a human being were lying alongside the skeleton of a cat: the two had been ceremoniously buried together and had rested undisturbed for 10,000 years.

Fewer than forty of those 10,000 years are represented in this book via the cats who inhabit vintage photographic postcards. For most collectors the Golden Age of the picture postcard extends from 1900 until the years of the First World War, but for those who seek out the privately made 'real photo' cards it has a second wind which lasts until the austerities of World War Two. Before the advent of photography, portraits of ordinary people, let alone their

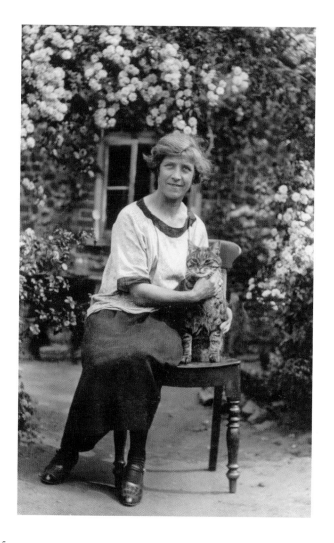

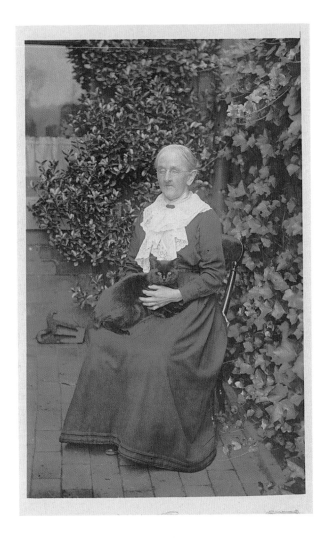

pets, were rare. The full democratisation of portraiture had to wait for the cheap and repeatable picture postcard. In the early years of the century, studios sprang up all over the world and a visit to the portrait photographer was no longer a luxury. Soon, it was not even a necessity as, with cheaper and faster film, it was possible to record the family's likeness on a bright day in the garden. This is where cats come into their own for, unlike dogs, they are reluctant travellers and recalcitrant sitters. In alien territory they hear the call of the wild and, even if basketed to the photographer's premises, cannot easily be persuaded to collude with strangers in a process that seems to bring them no benefit. Hence the majority of family cats are photographed in customary places or on familiar laps. Even so, the cat is not to be meddled with and is unwilling to be cradled in arms or to be held aloft for the camera for too long. The furry-edged streak or stripy blur of an escaping cat is a feature of many garden portraits.

In the studios of commercial publishers all is different. Specialised photogenic and photogenial cats here go through their paces on home ground and may offer several poses in a session (p. 42). The resulting pictures, tuned to a largely sentimental market, were made in their millions, often with mawkish captions which, it must be confessed, have occasionally been masked in the more saccharine of the examples presented in this book. Tinting, either mechanical or hand done (mostly by women at almost slave labour rates) was a frequent extra with colours from the sugared almond range.

The antics of kittens provided endless possibilities. Curiosity may not have killed the cat but it certainly commercialised the kittens. The provision of any prop on a table would instantly have a group of kittens playing round it. As they explored a basket or examined a hat, the camera would be ready to click and, when they tumbled in, the publisher's wordsmith would be thinking of a caption along the lines of *A brimful of trouble*.

At the posh end of the feline glamour industry are the continental, mostly French, cards which aspire to the style and finish of Salon oil paintings with artful juxtapositions of pretty girl and pampered animal.

Yet such images, for all their artifice, cunning

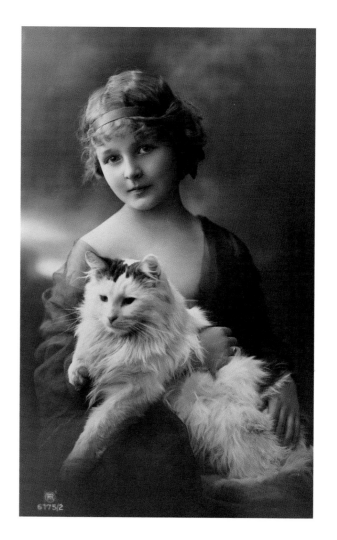

7

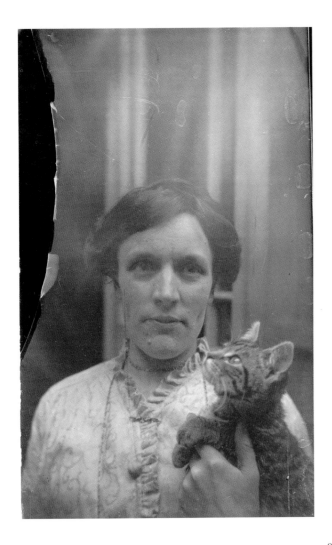

lighting and subsequent touch with the airbrush, do not quite provoke the same emotional engagement as the real vernacular cat in a robustly real environment with a real, relevant and unberibboned person. The half blind old lady (p. 6) with her cat on her lap, its eyes large enough to serve for two, belongs to a narrative world which has an authentic past and an imaginable future. Even lower down the scale of apparent artistry, this card (*left*), from a broken negative, of a plain woman with a plain tabby cat, asks a more mysterious question. What was it that made this image, despite its damage and unflattering directness, call for rescue and perpetuity?

Although this book deals with pictures that derive from photographs, the majority of cat postcards were drawn by artists. The most celebrated of these, Louis Wain, makes a guest appearance in the dream of a handsome studio cat (p. 93). Cartoon cats were also common and they find their way into these pages via the huge novelty dolls of Felix that were the popular draws of Margate's beach photographers.

The element of caricature is present here when it serves some real purpose, as in the cat (p. 79) recruited to promote the suffragette movement and sport the colours of emancipation.

Most of the cats in these pages are anonymous, although a name is sometimes scrawled on the back or mentioned in a message. Some of the people, however, are, or were, well known. Except for the occasional literary figure like Collette (p. 127) they are mostly the music-hall performers of the time like the Dare sisters, or wonderfully obscure film stars like Heather Angel (p. 137). Most notorious is the chorus girl Evelyn Nesbit (p. 44) who, as the wife of playboy and killer Harry Thaw, had a real-life role in a famous murder trial. Celebrities amongst cats themselves were the ships' mascots, one of whom is seen curled up in the barrel mouth of a huge naval gun.

Since this present compilation is a companion book to Libby Hall's *Postcard Dogs*, it should not come as a surprise to see some interbreeding in the form of an occasional dog who sneaks in (albeit chaperoned by a cat). This is no fluke since dogs and cats seem to get on very well together without treading on each other's paws. Cats even seem to be more patient sitters for the camera when a dog is present,

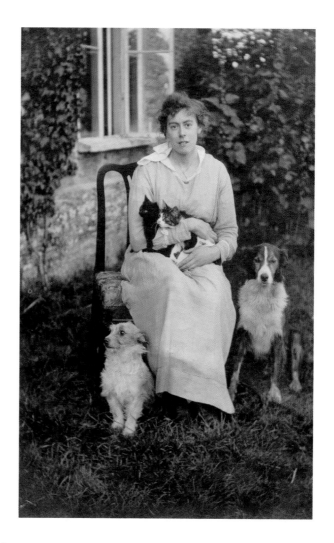

as if the dog gives some sort of osmotic reassurance to the instinctively mistrustful cat.

The virtue that sets cats apart from dogs is that (except as mouse-catchers) they are sublimely useless. They pull no arctic sledges and deliver no brandy to stranded mountaineers, nor do they guide, nor sniff out drugs, although I'm sure that their noses are as sensitive. Their role is to be the exemplar of the animal kingdom in our midst; real beasts, lone hunters who once outside the house are tigers in their territory.

All these cats are long since dead as, with the exception of an odd centenarian, are their protectors (since one can hardly be said to own a cat). Even some of the photographs have started to fade away: the lady below is happy with her cats, enjoying the stoical watchfulness of one and the pleasure of feeding the other. This cat moment, like so many presented in the following pages, has been preserved and the card itself arrested on its journey towards pale sepia oblivion. Owner, pet and image thus survive as another memento of that strange bond between the feline and the human animal which can be trusted to last another 10,000 years.

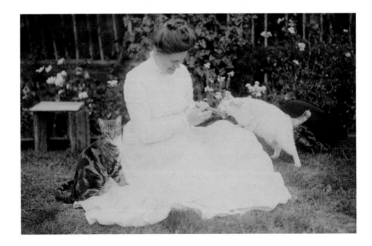

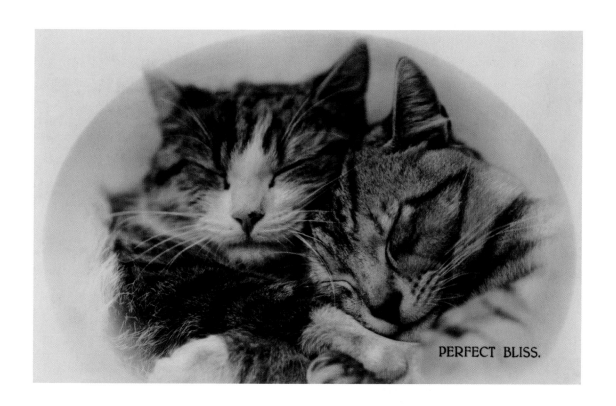

PERFECT BLISS.

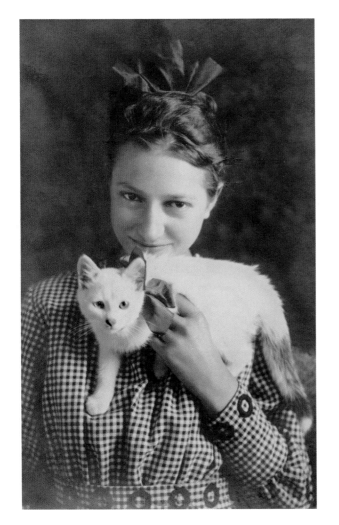
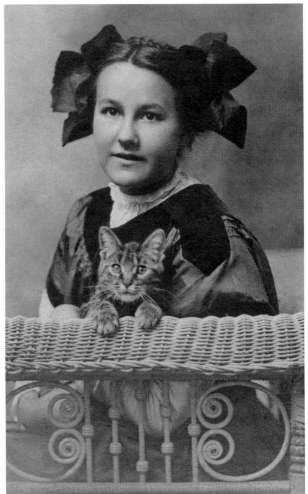

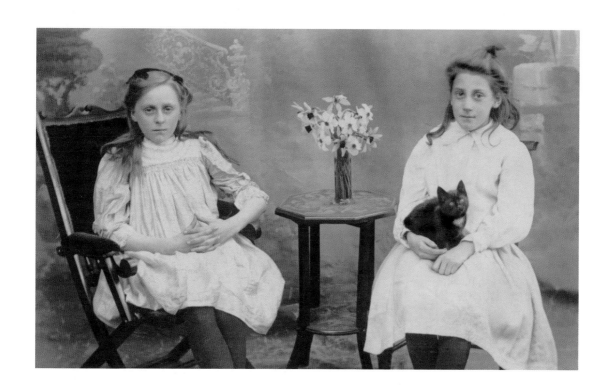

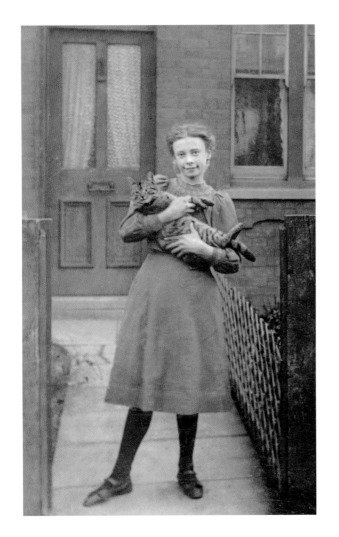

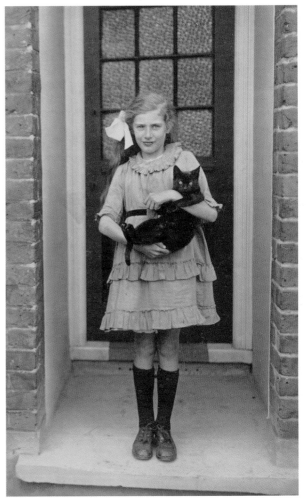

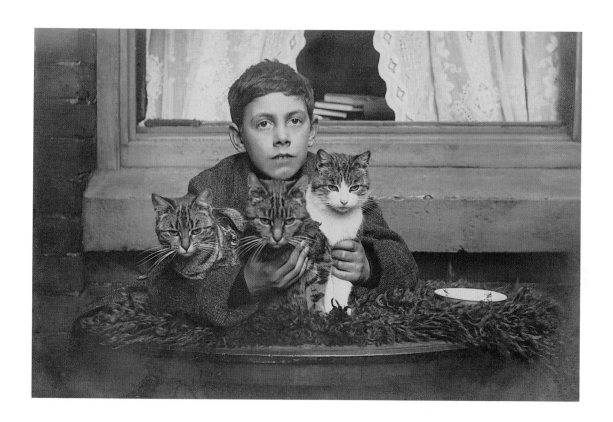

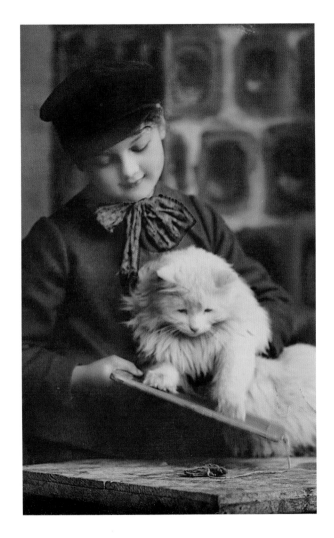

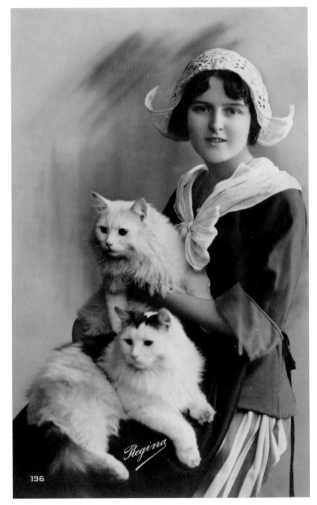

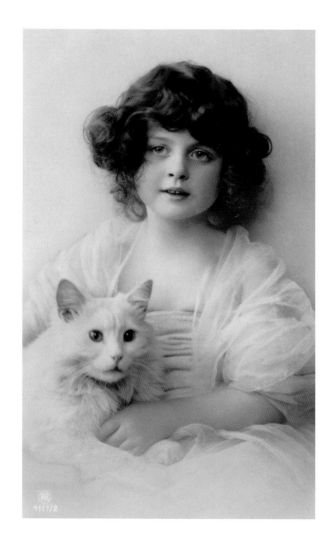
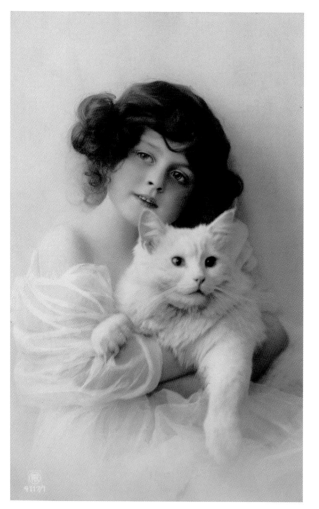

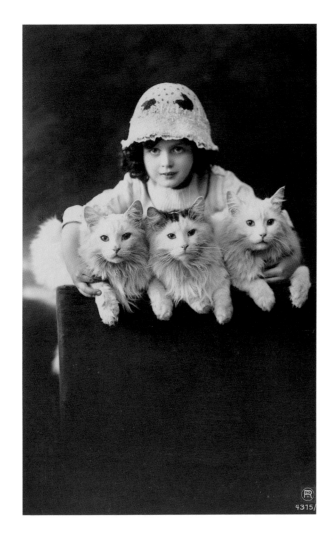

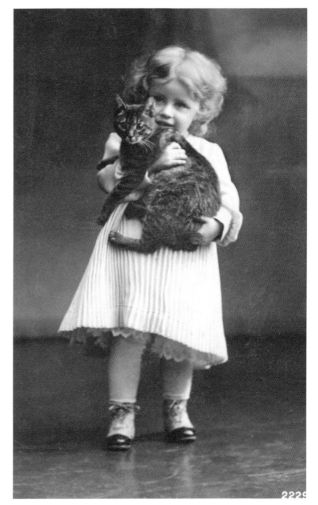

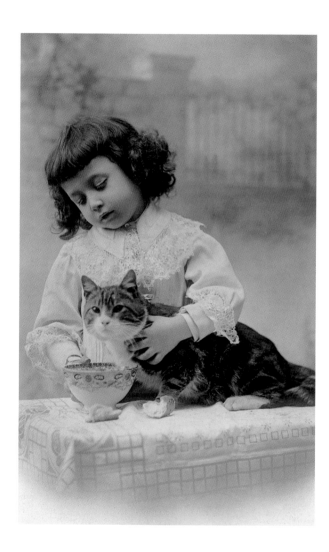

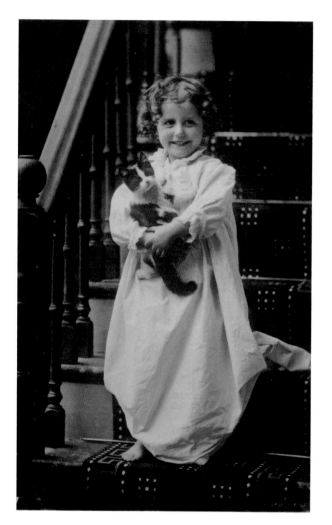

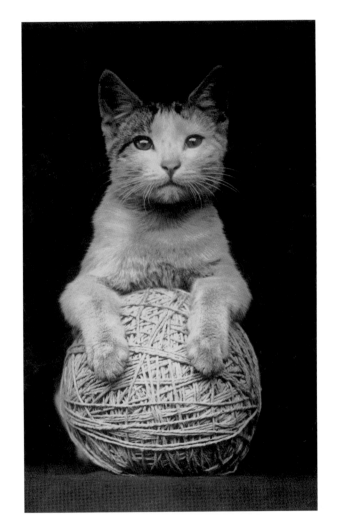

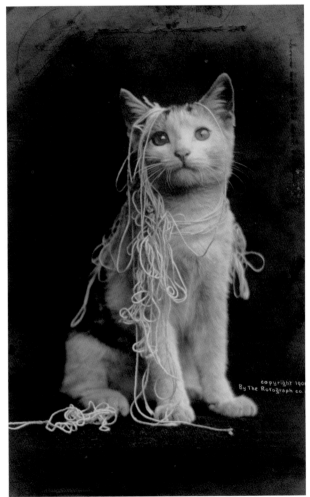

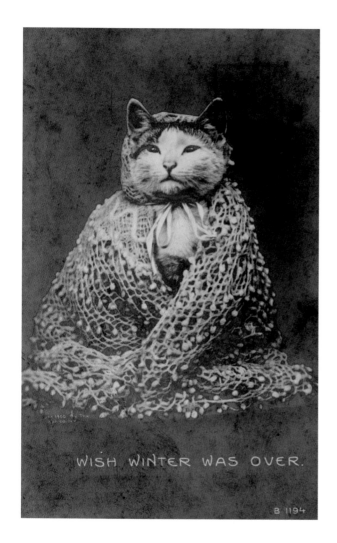

WISH WINTER WAS OVER.

B 1194

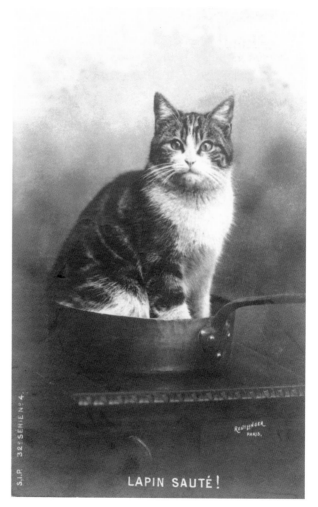

LAPIN SAUTÉ !

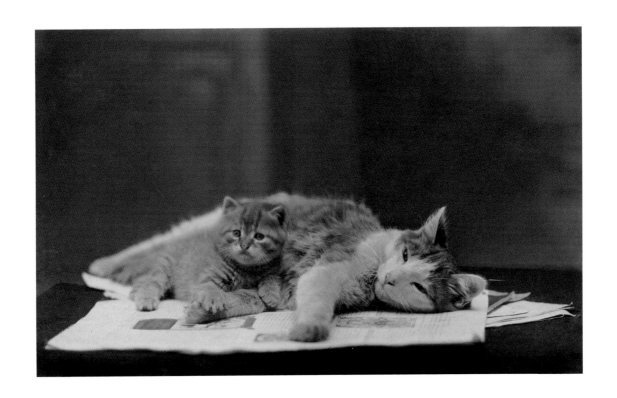

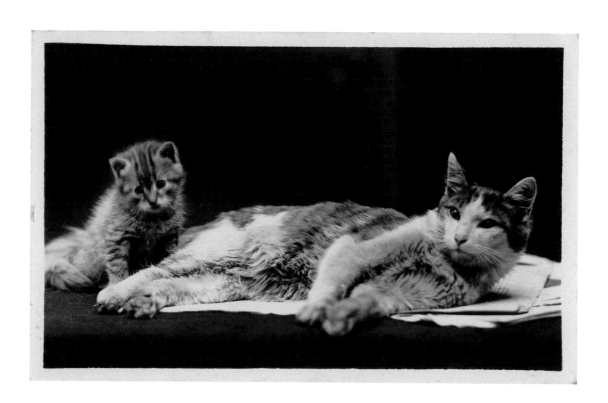

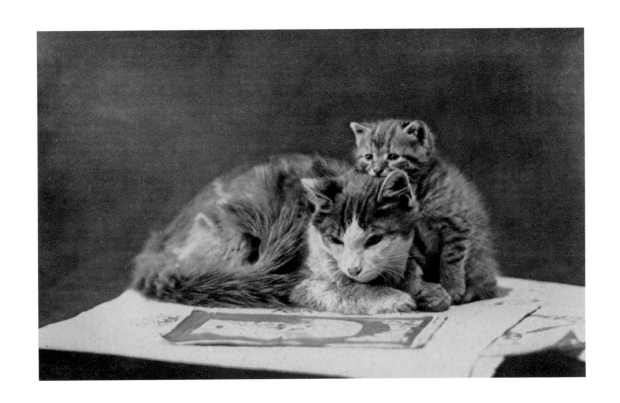

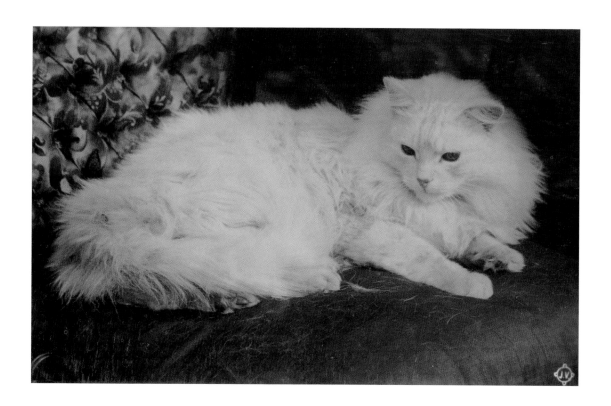

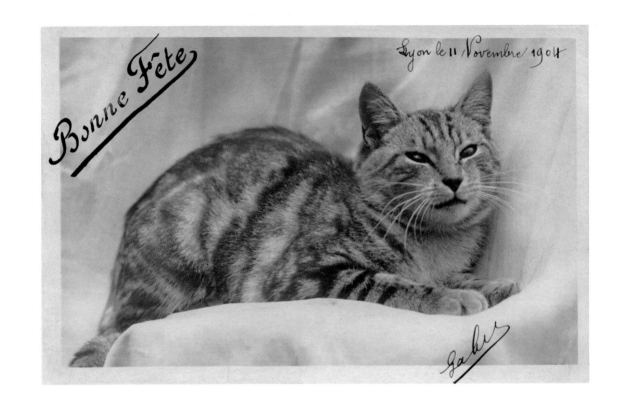

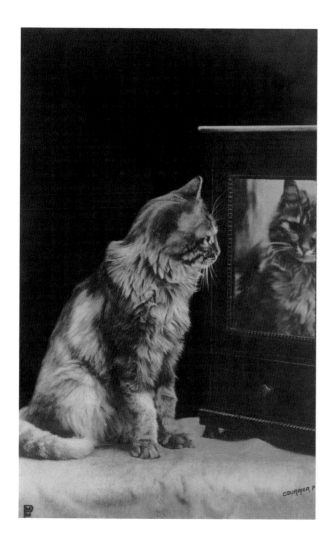

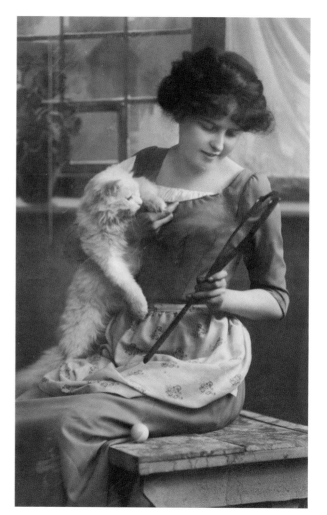

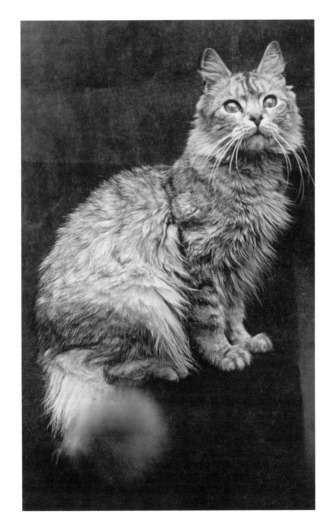
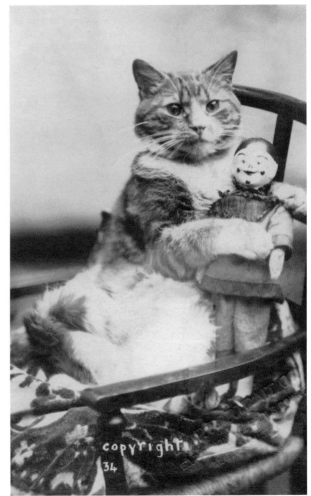

copyright
34

28

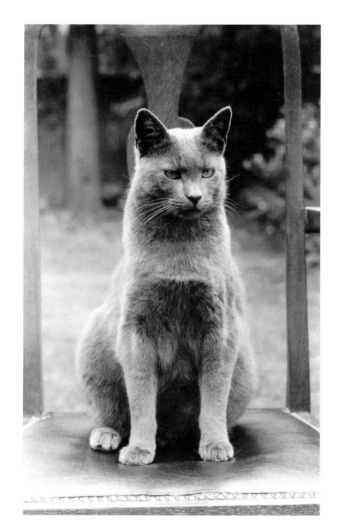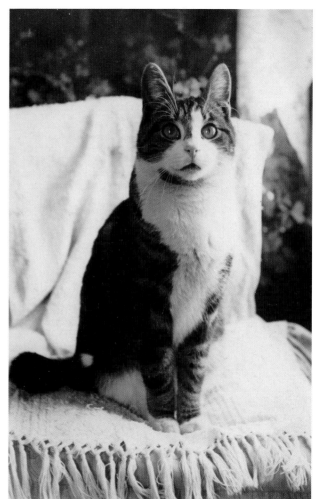

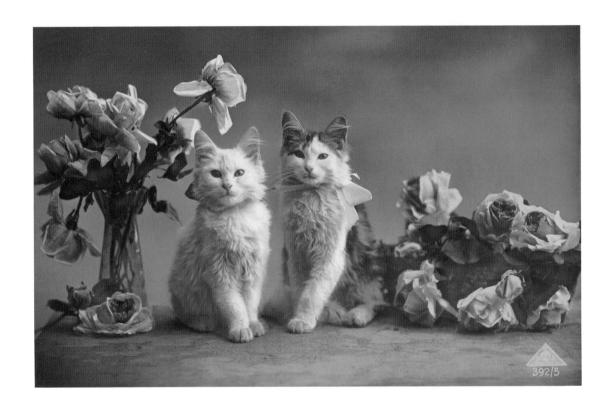

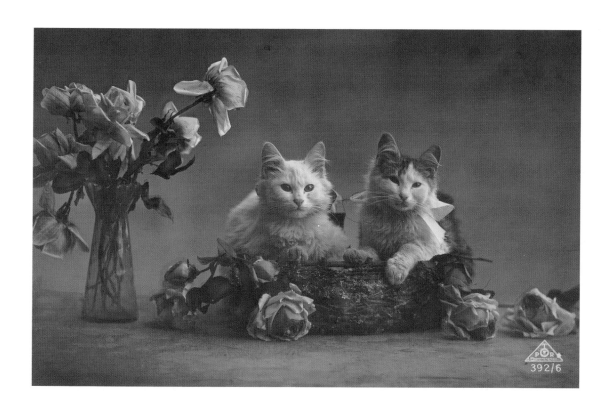

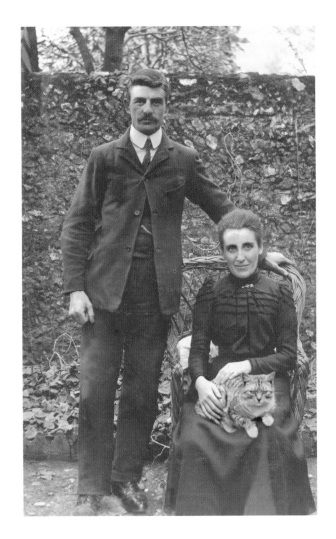

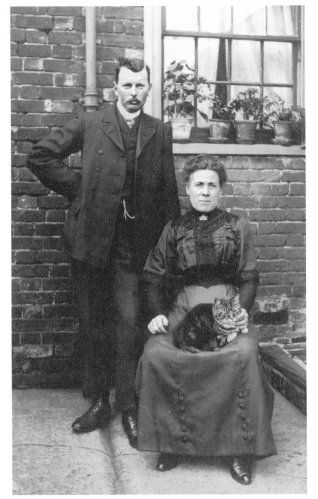

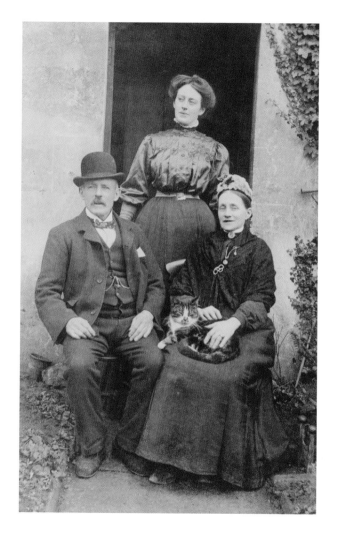

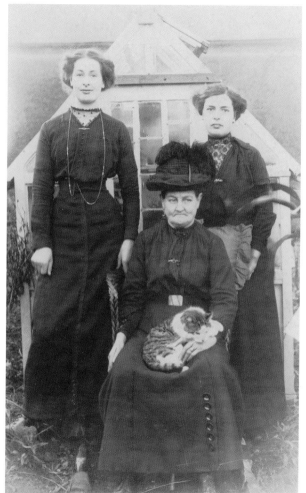

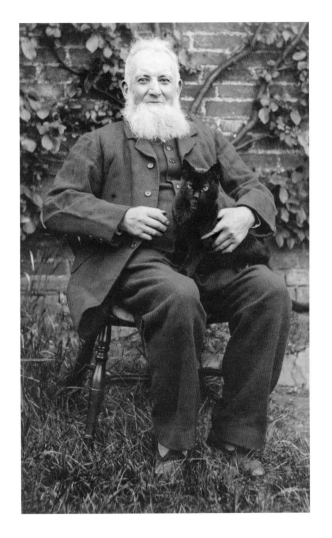

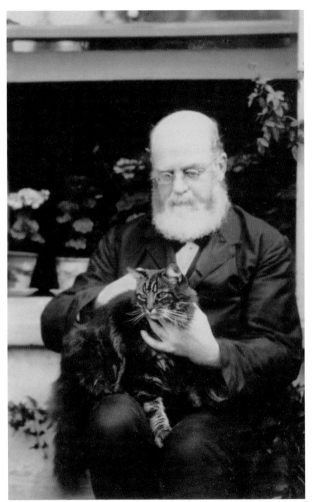

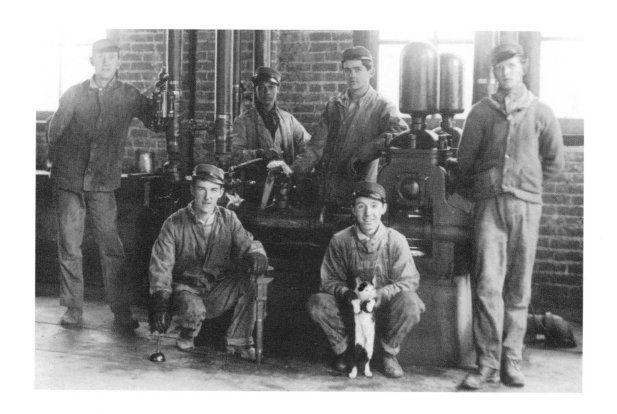

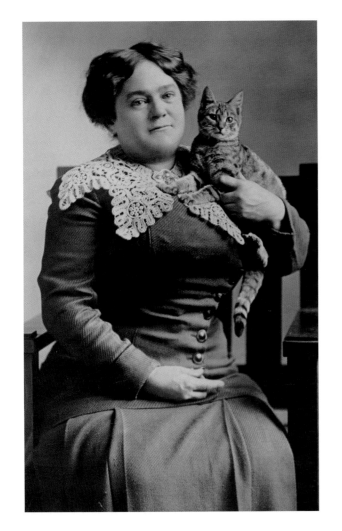

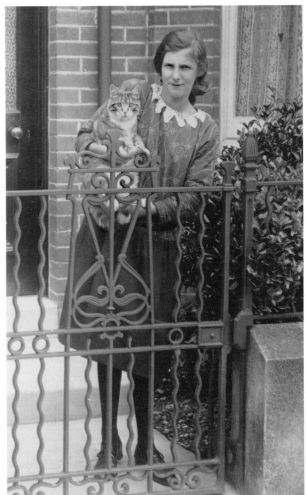

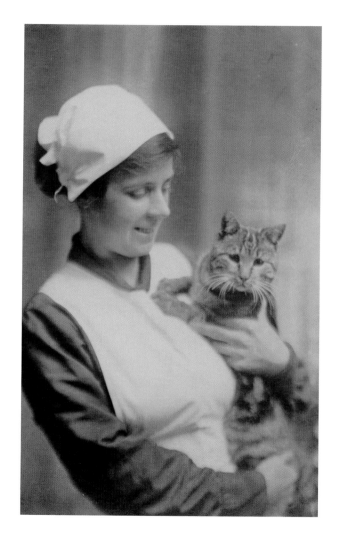

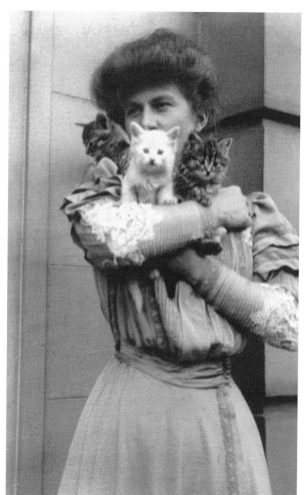

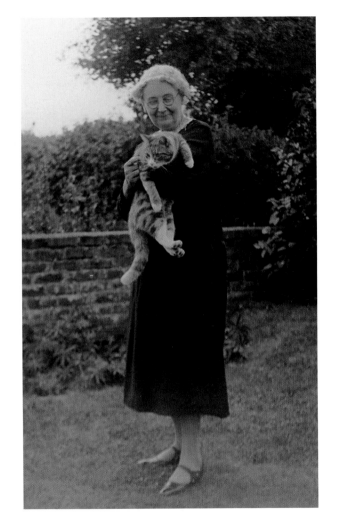
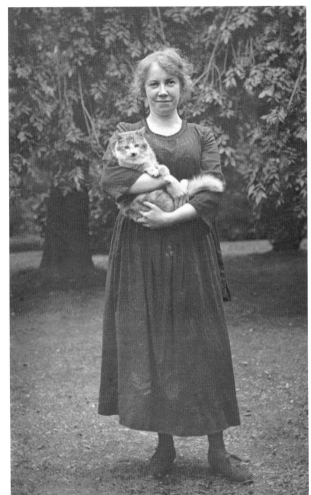

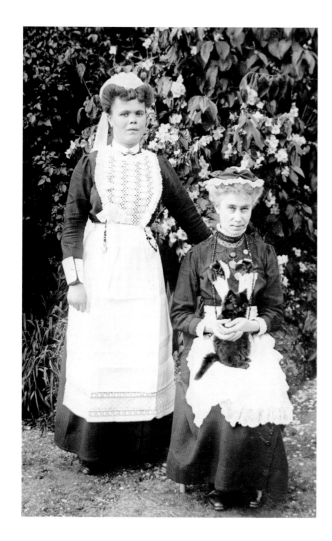

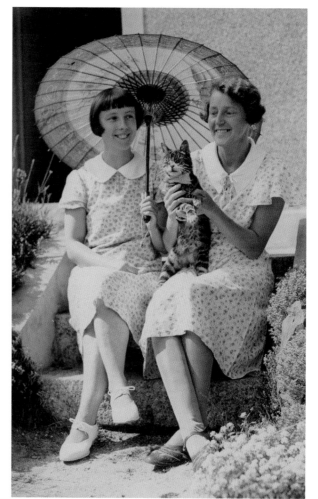

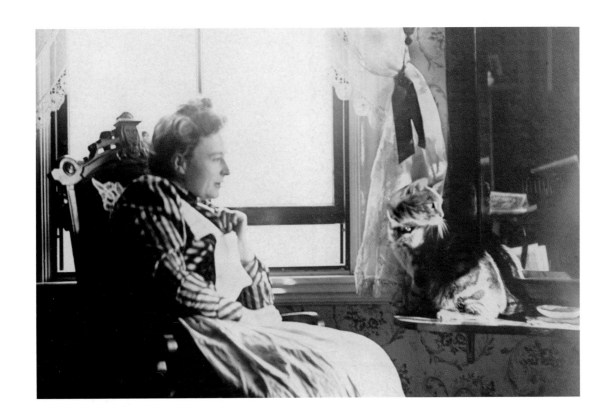

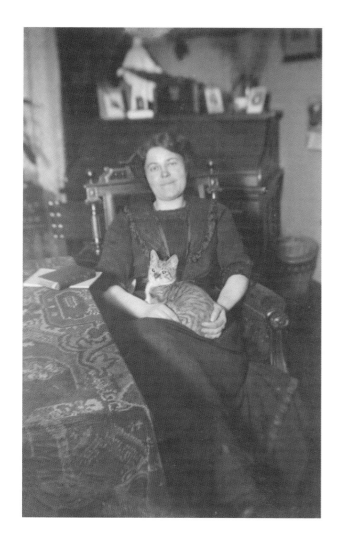
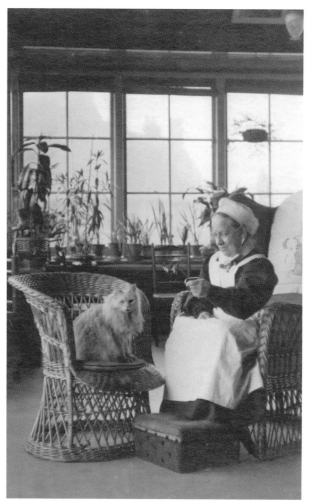

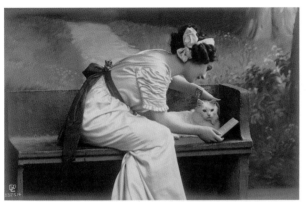

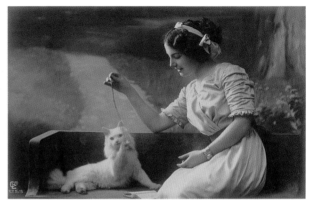

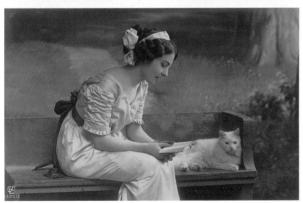

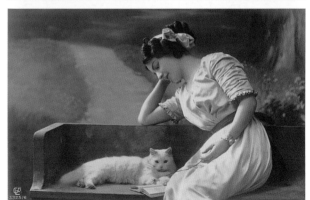

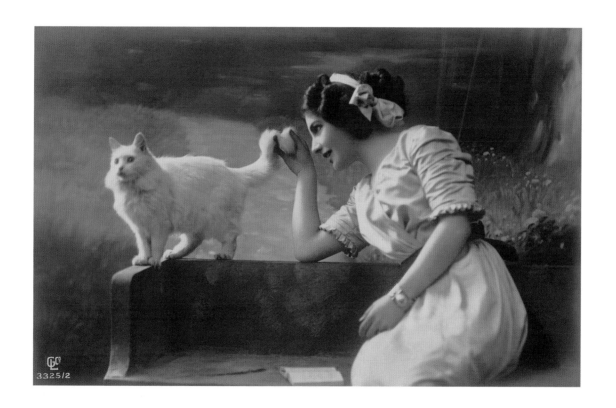

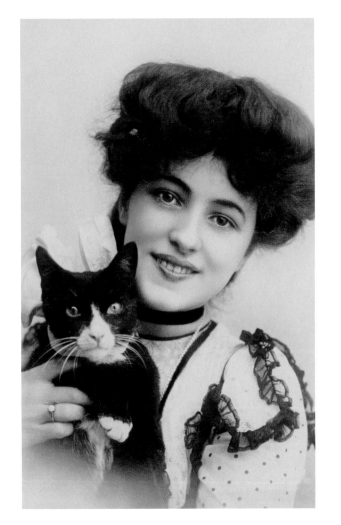

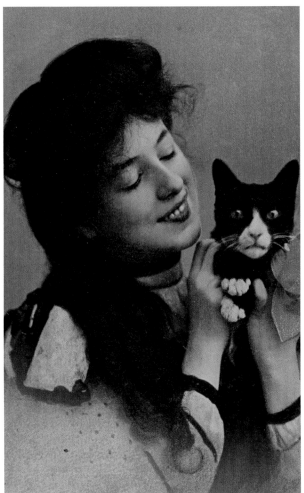

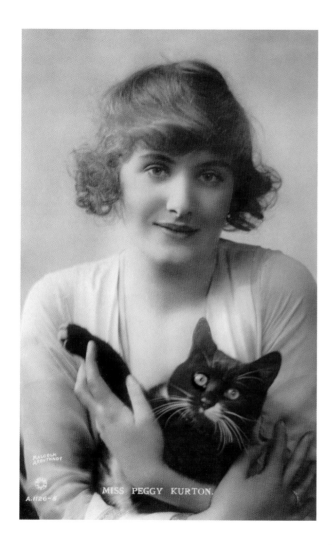

MISS PEGGY KURTON.

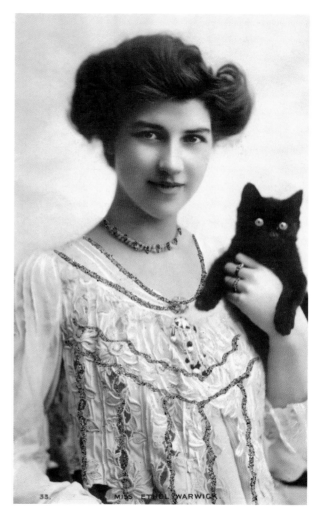

MISS ETHEL WARWICK.

45

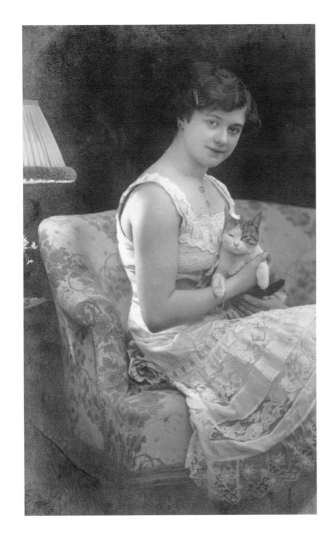 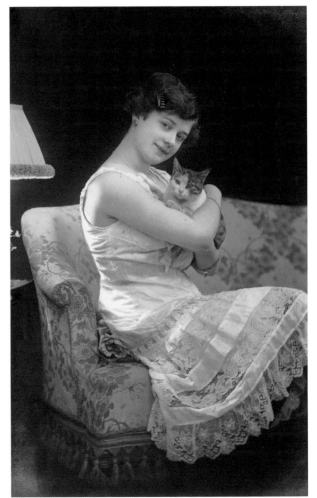

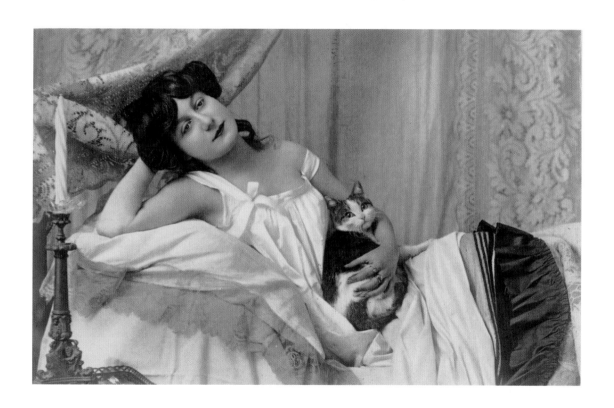

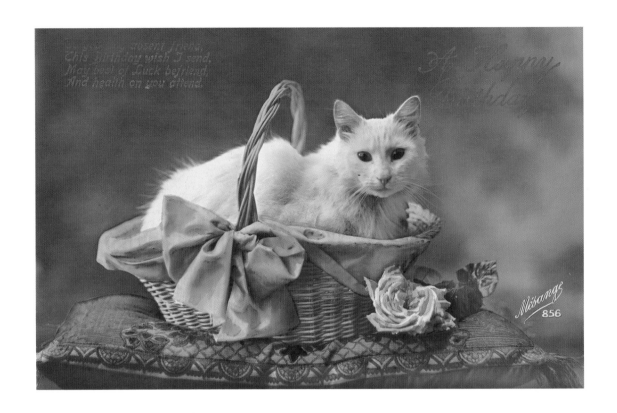

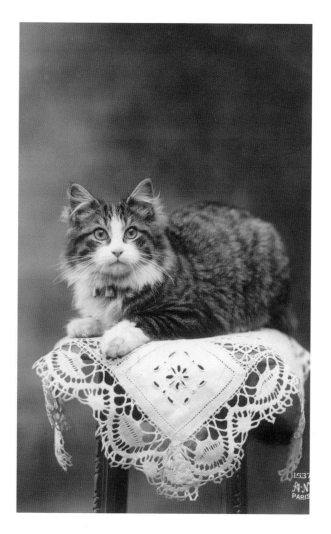

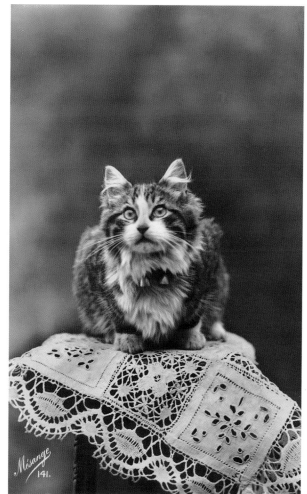

49

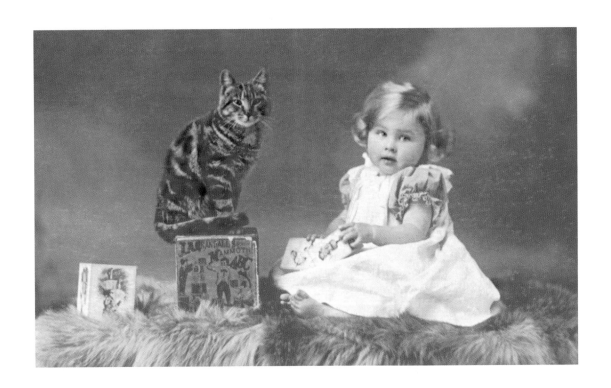

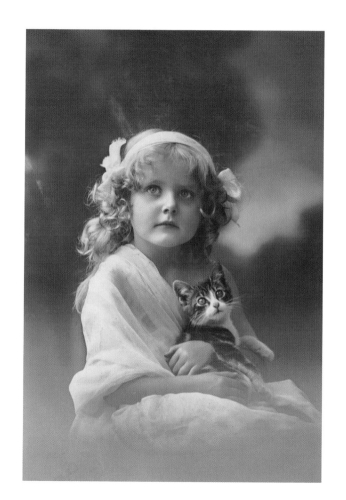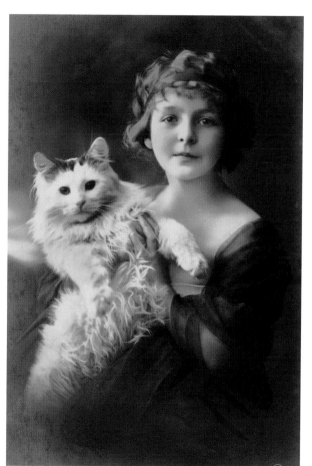

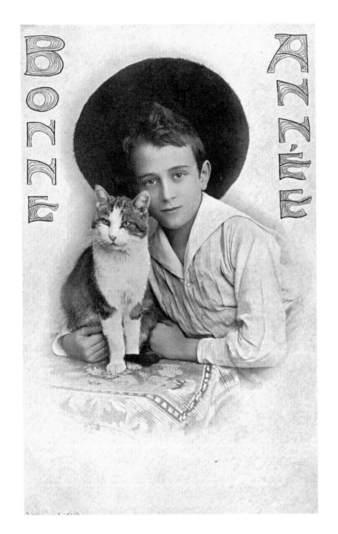

BONNE ANNÉE

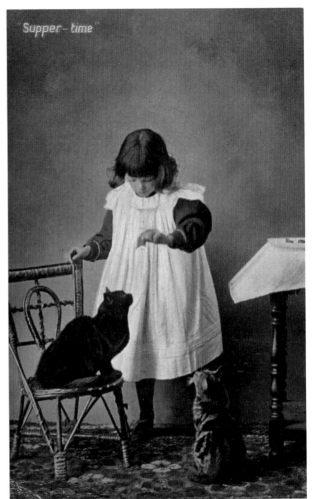

"Supper-time"

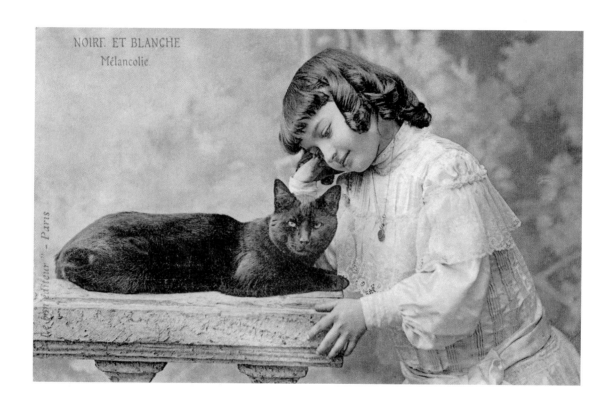

NOIRE ET BLANCHE
Mélancolie.

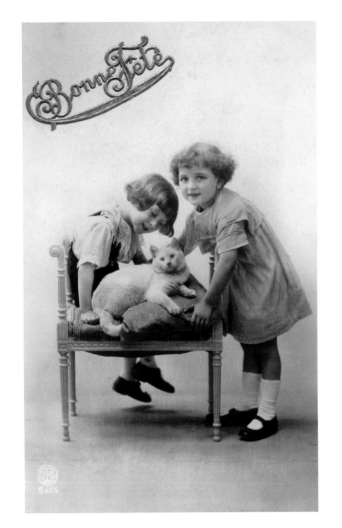

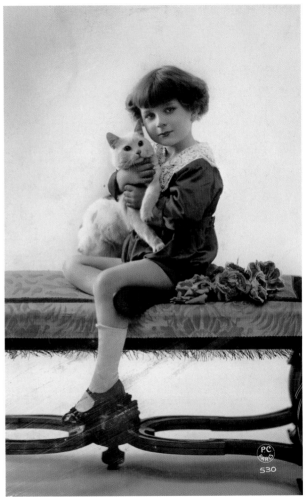

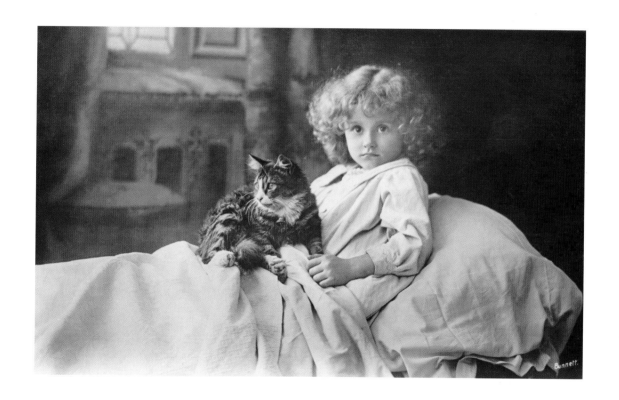

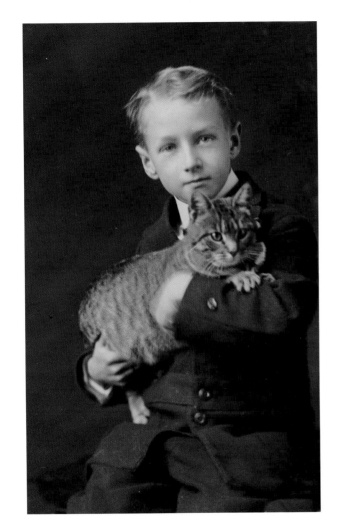
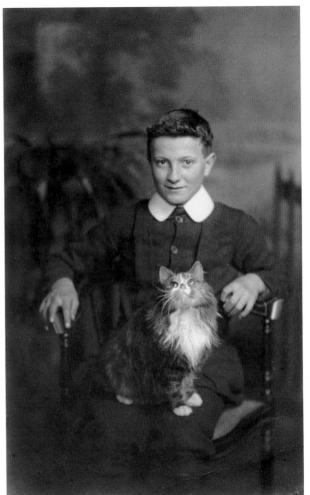

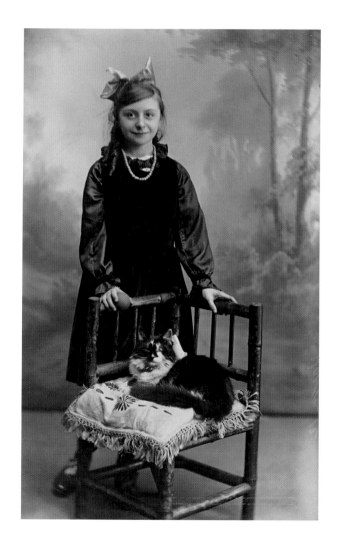

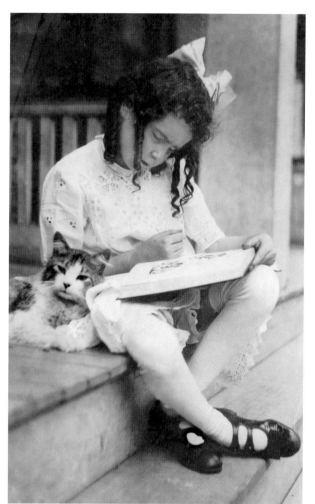

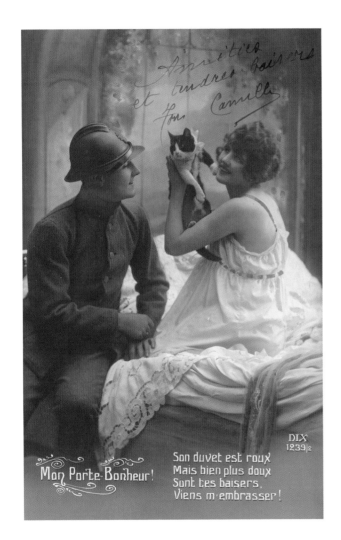

Amitiés
et tendres baisers
Ton Camille

DLX
1239/2

Mon Porte-Bonheur!

Son duvet est roux
Mais bien plus doux
Sont tes baisers,
Viens m'embrasser!

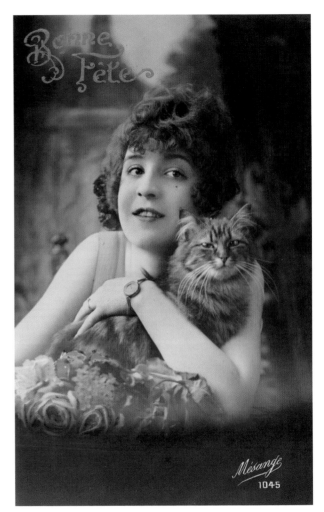

Bonne Fête

Mésange
1045

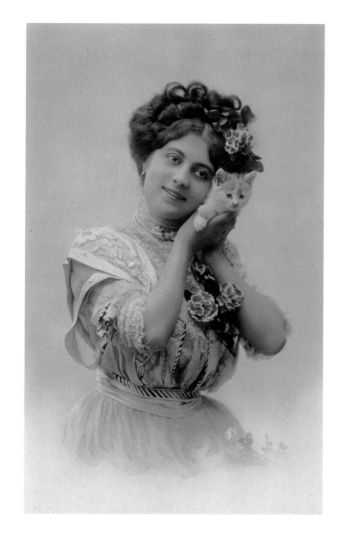

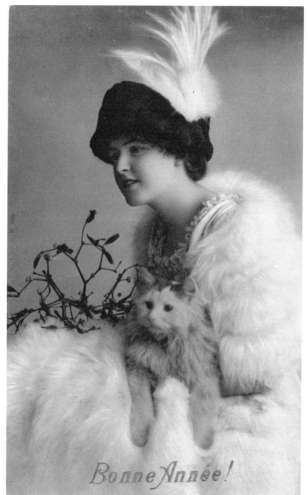

Bonne Année!

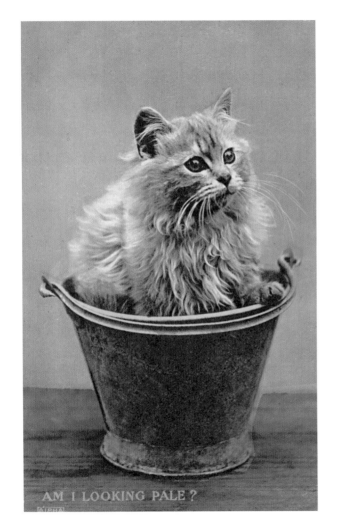

AM I LOOKING PALE?

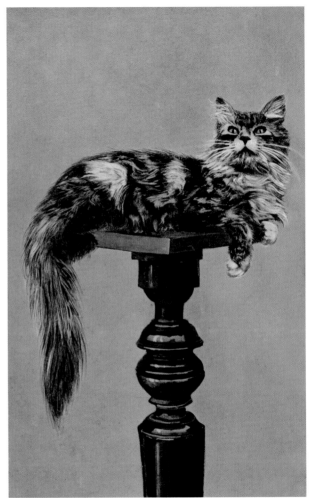

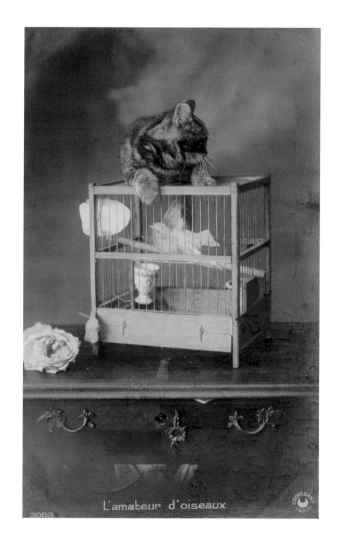

L'amateur d'oiseaux

3083

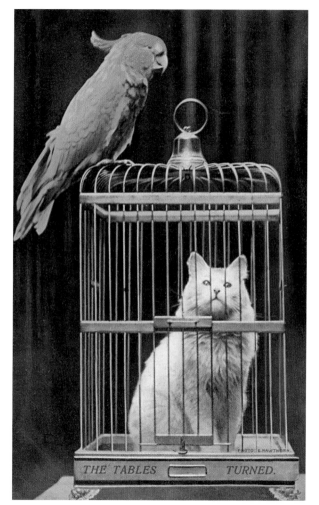

THE TABLES TURNED.

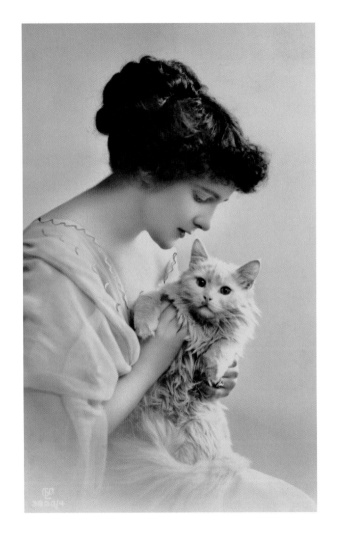

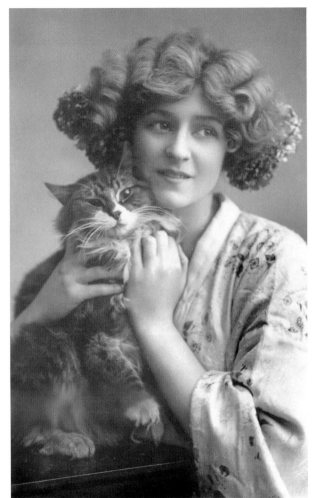

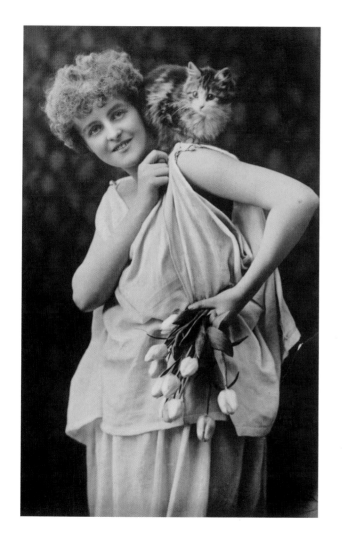

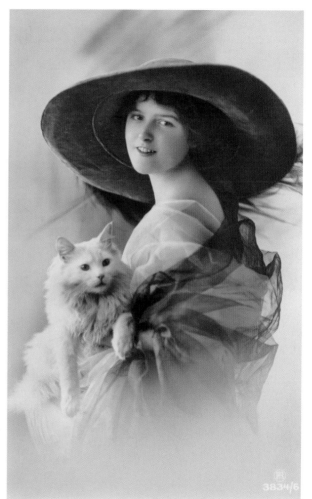

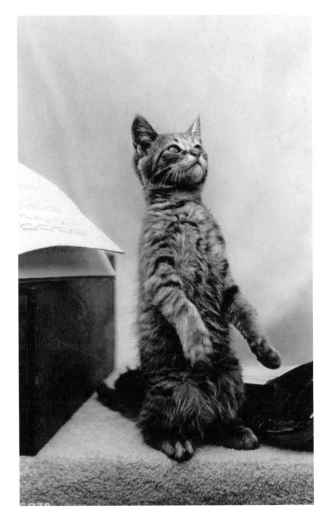

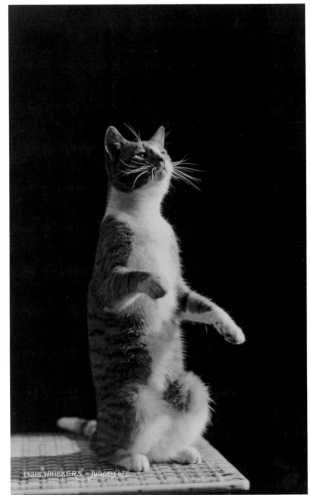

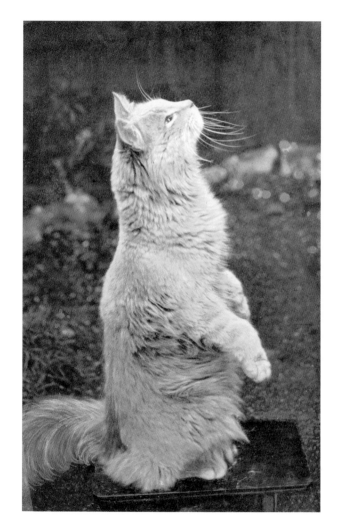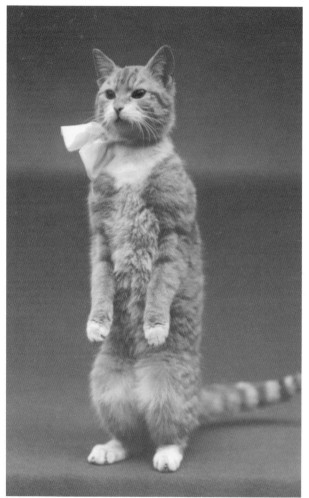

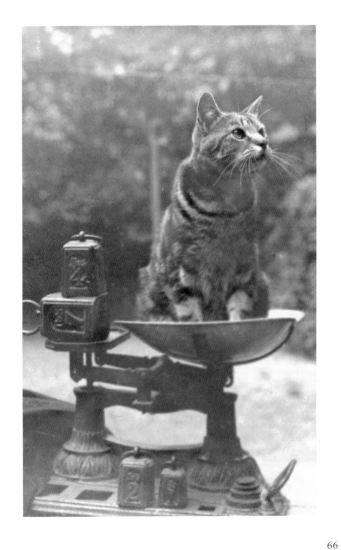

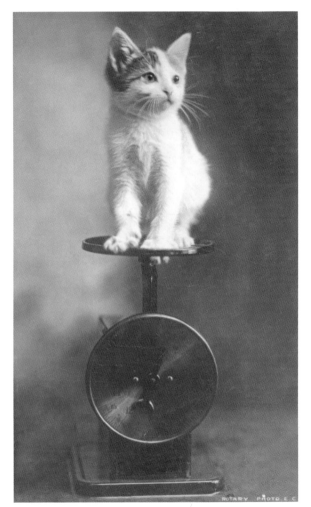

66

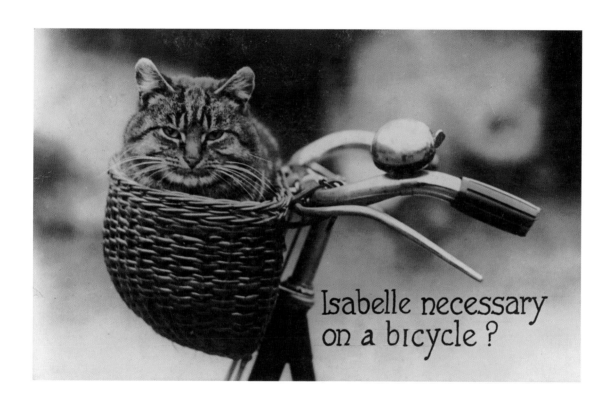

Isabelle necessary on a bicycle?

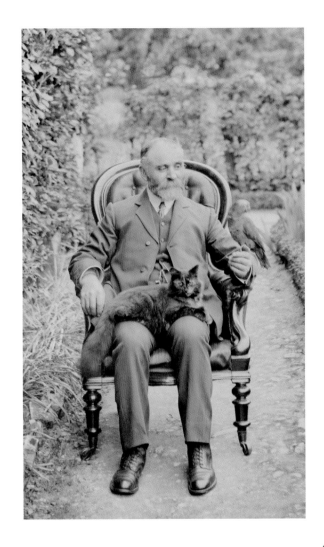

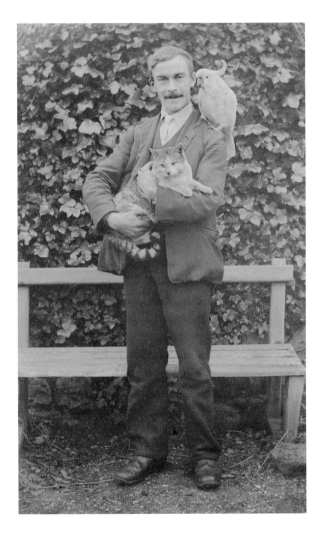

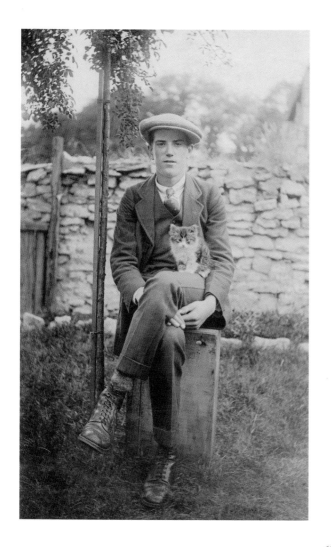

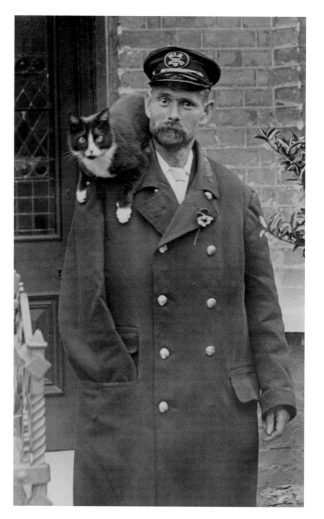

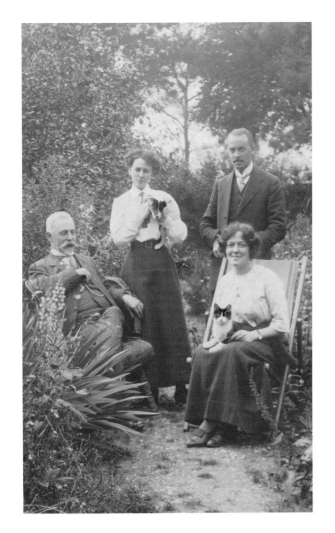

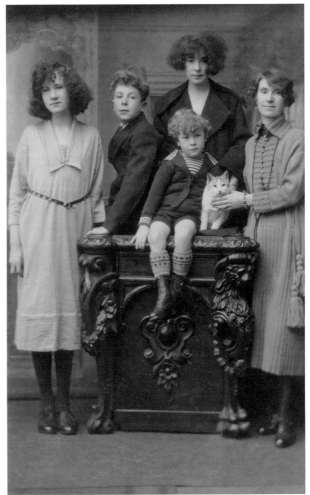

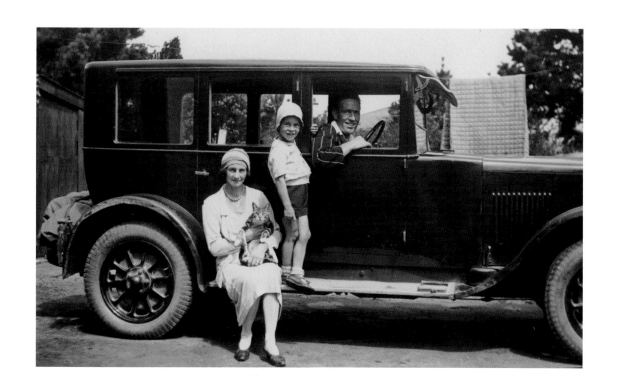

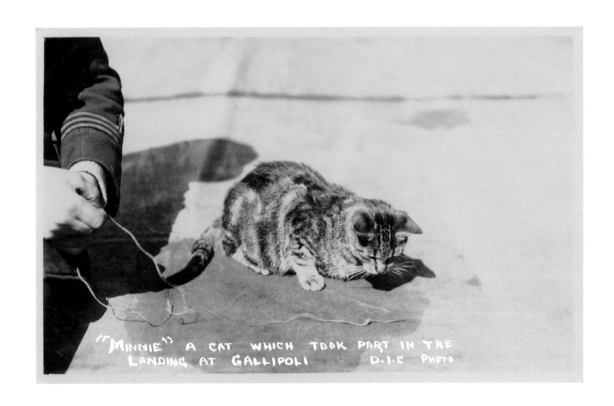

"Minnie" a cat which took part in the landing at Gallipoli   D.I.C Photo

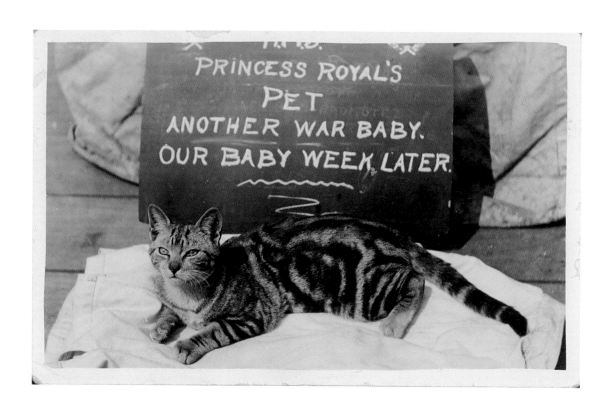

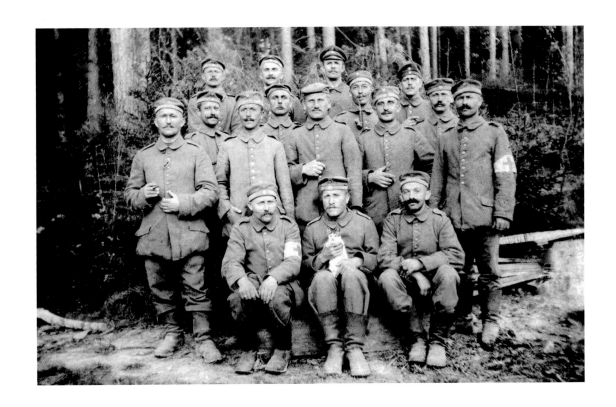

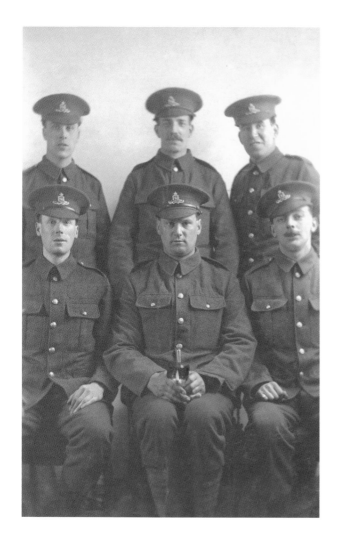

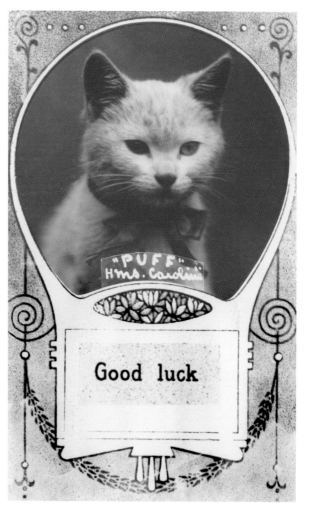

"PUFF"
Hms. Caroline

Good luck

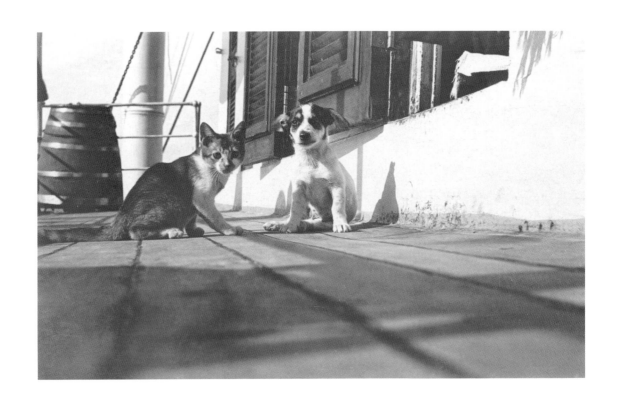

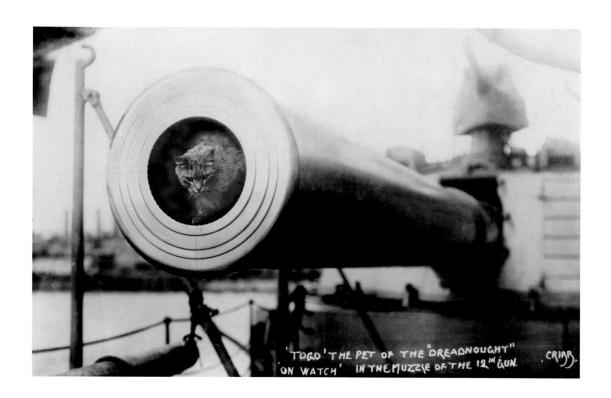

'TOGO' THE PET OF THE "DREADNOUGHT"
'ON WATCH' IN THE MUZZLE OF THE 12 IN GUN. ·CRIBB·

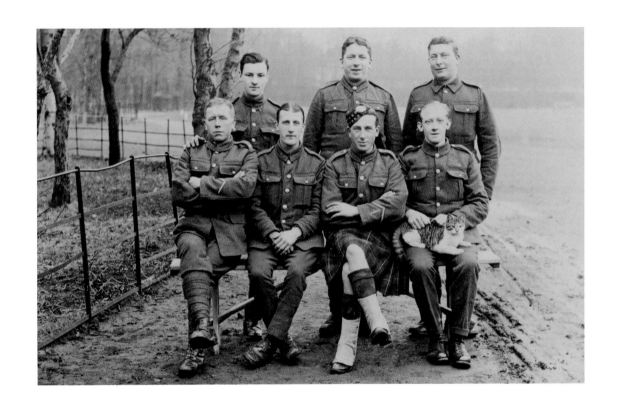

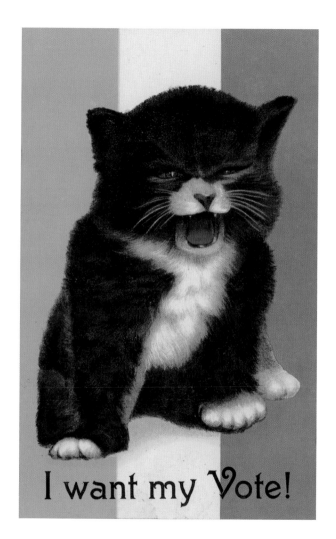

I want my Vote!

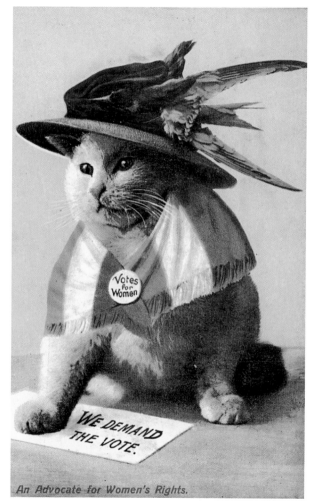

Votes for Women

WE DEMAND THE VOTE.

An Advocate for Women's Rights.

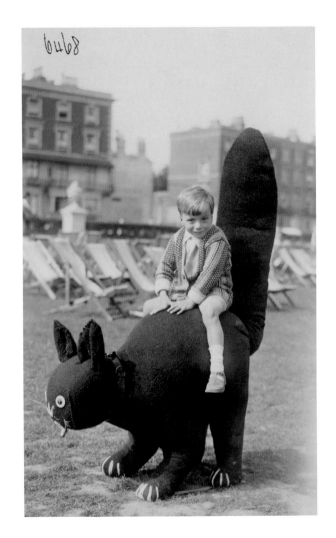

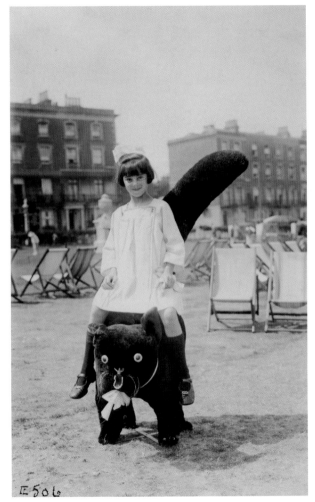

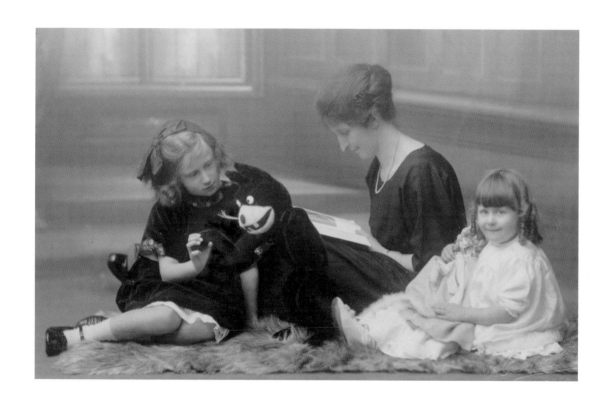

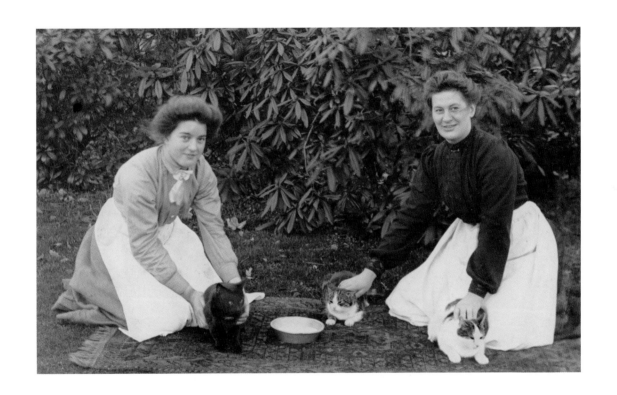

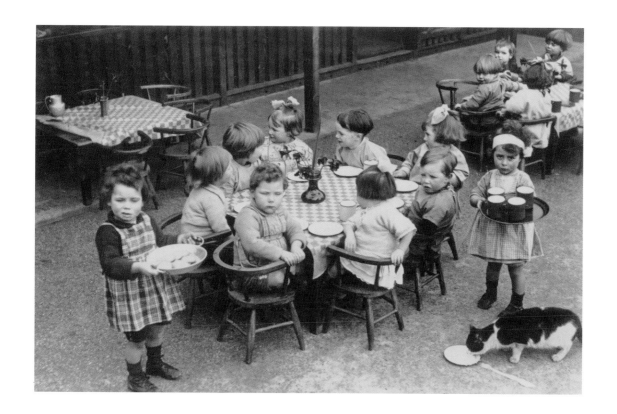

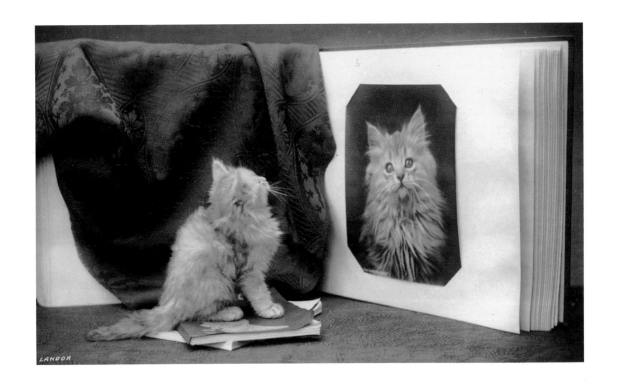

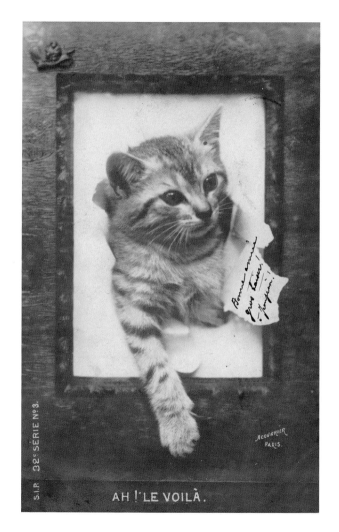

AH ! LE VOILÀ.

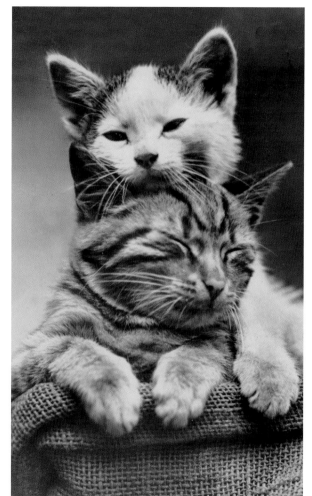

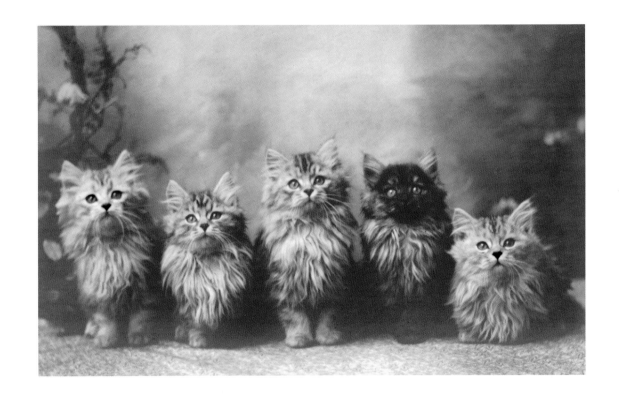

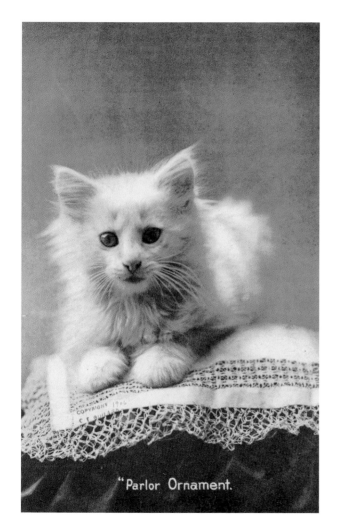

"Parlor Ornament.

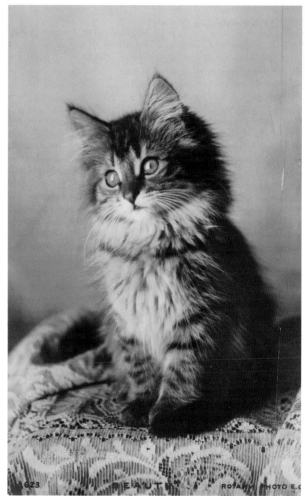

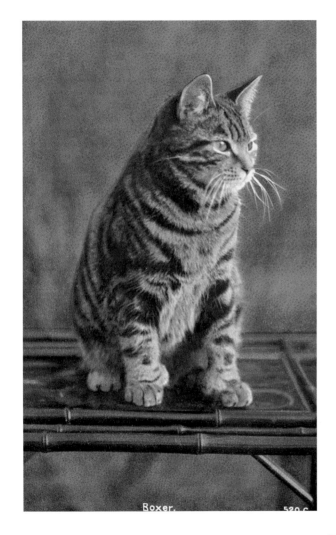

Boxer.

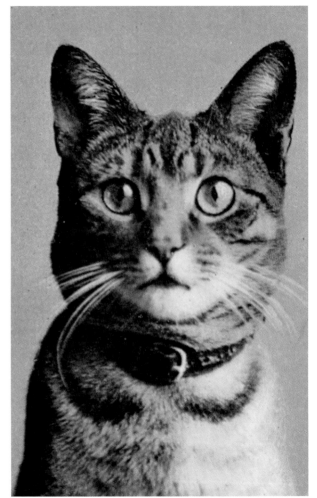

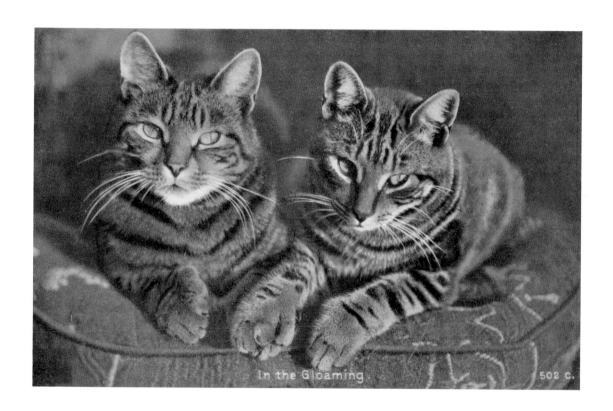

In the Gloaming.   502 c.

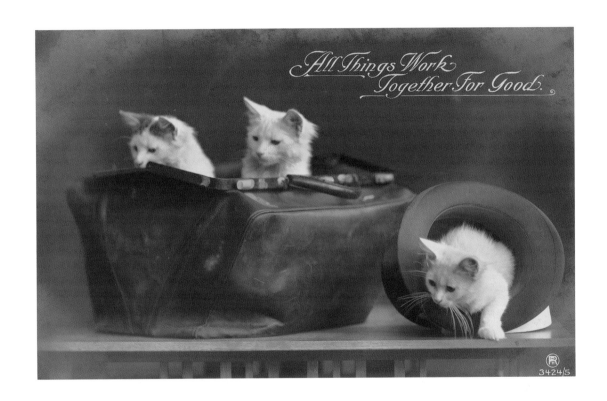

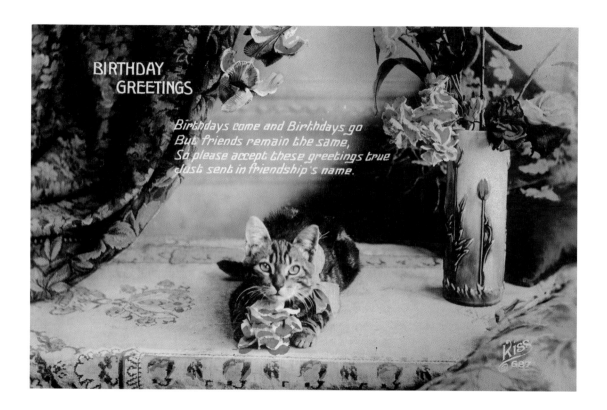

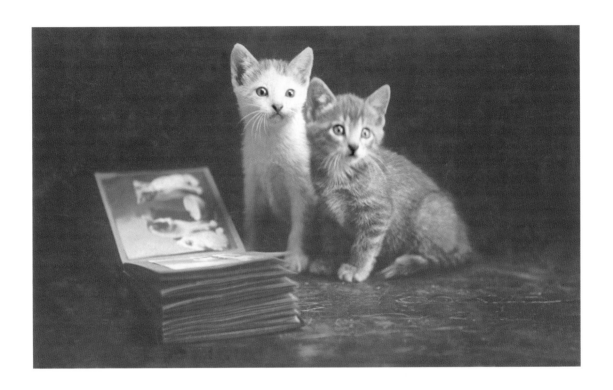

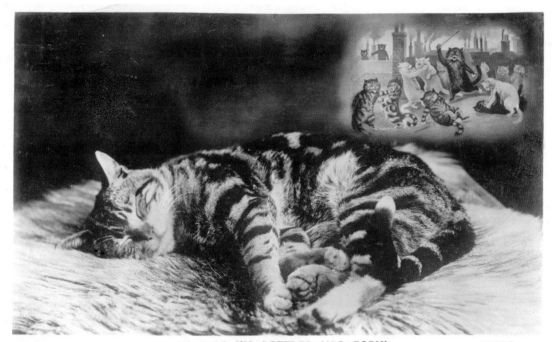

FIGHTING HIS BATTLES O'ER AGAIN.

950.L.

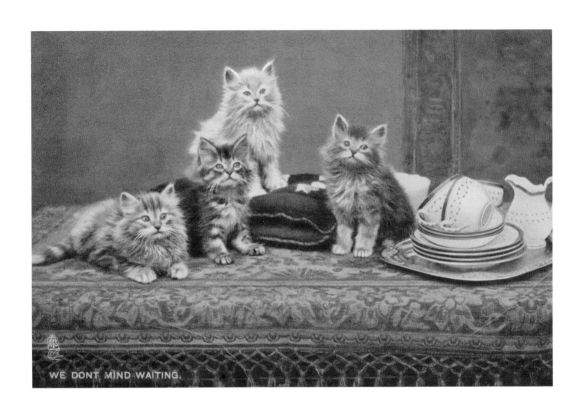

WE DON'T MIND WAITING.

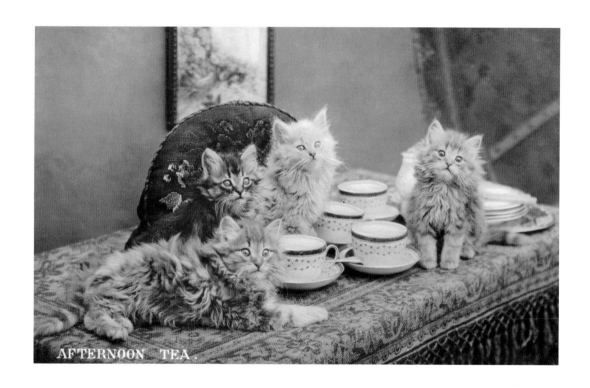

AFTERNOON TEA.

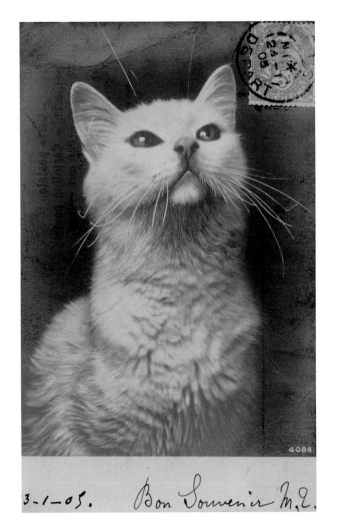

3-1-05. Bon Souvenir M.E.

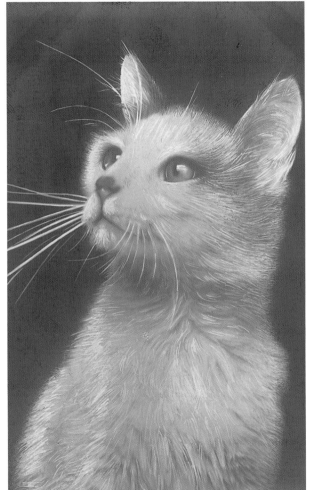

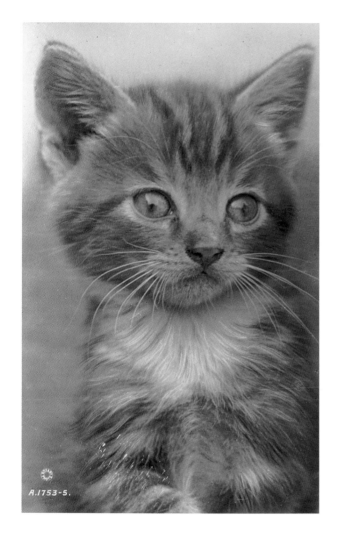

A.1753-5.

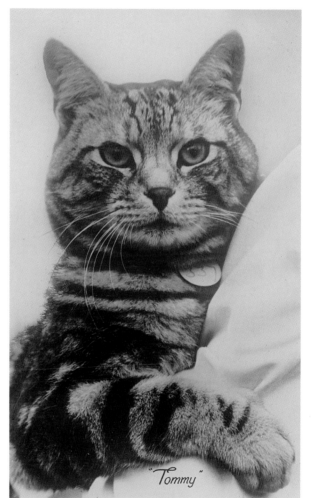

"Tommy"

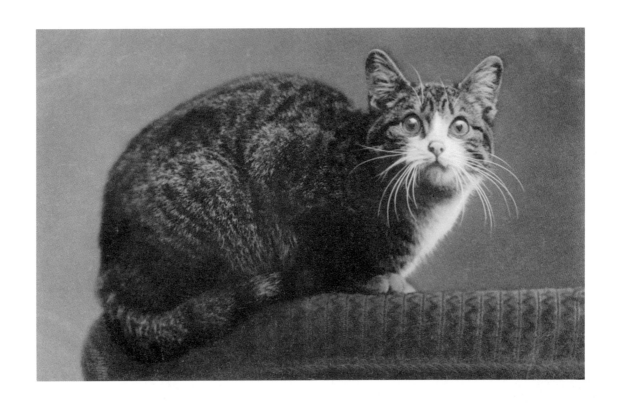

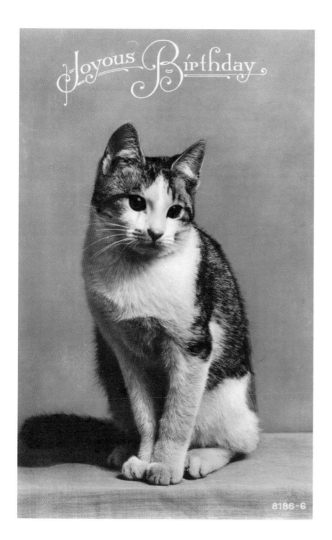

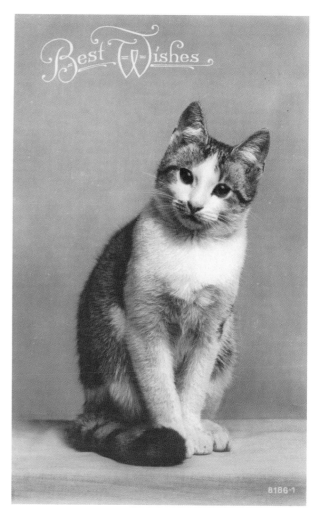

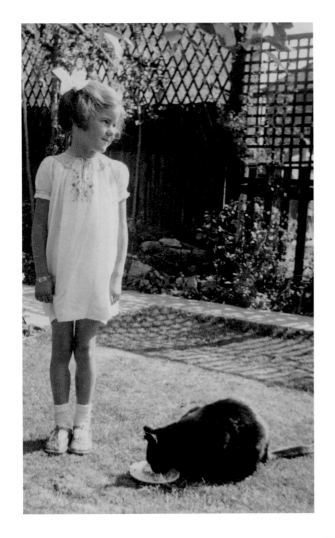

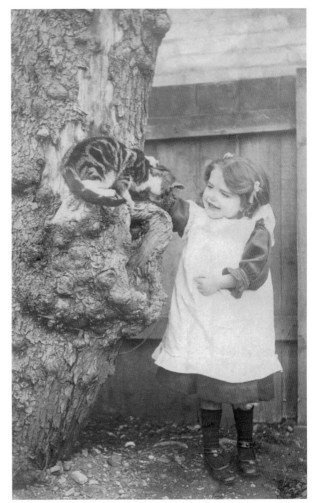

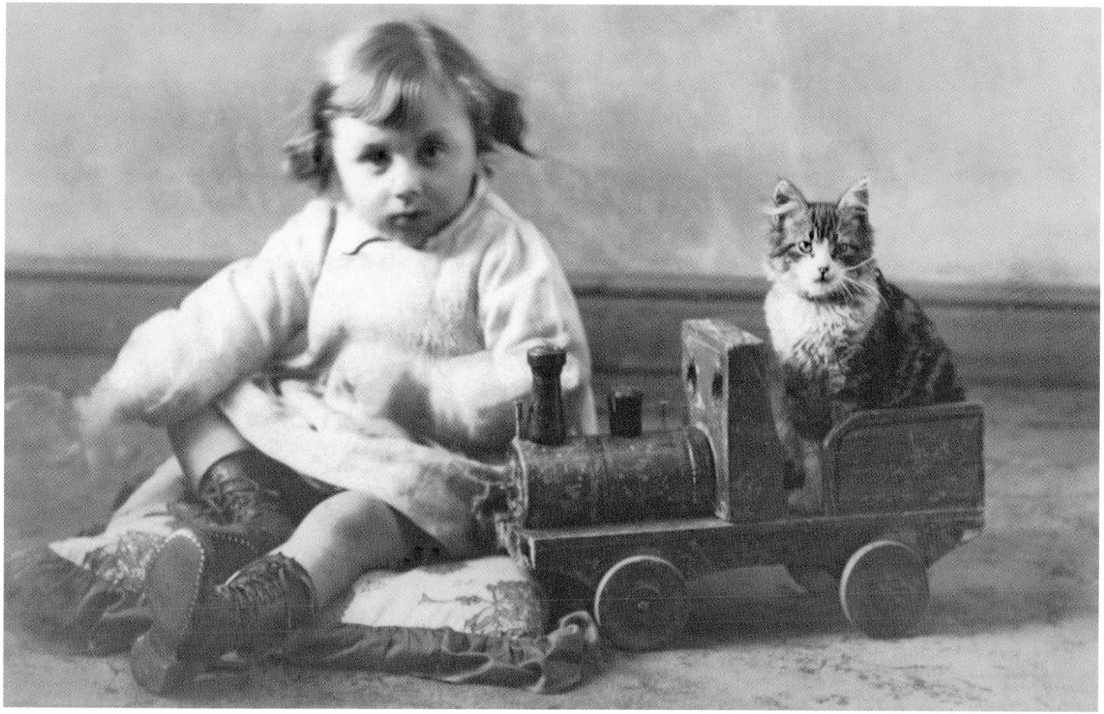

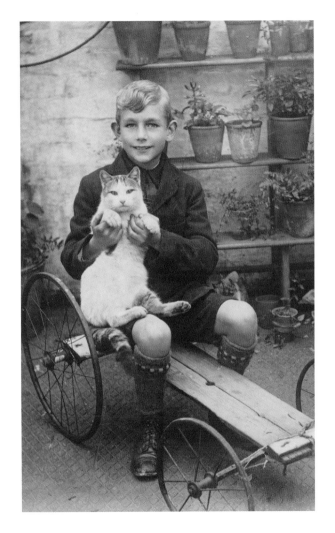

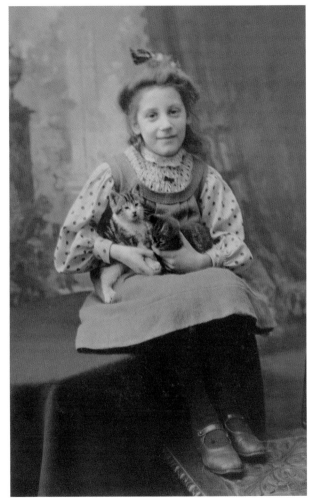

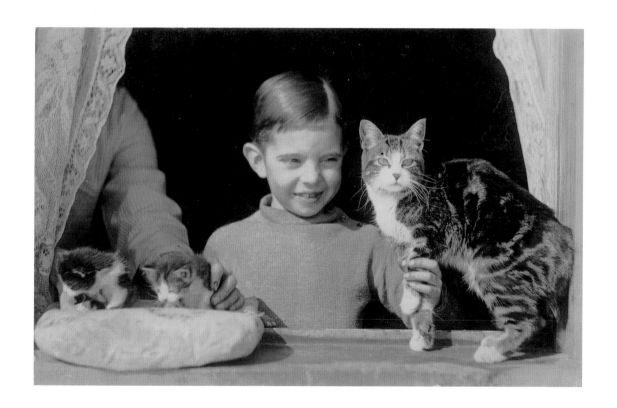

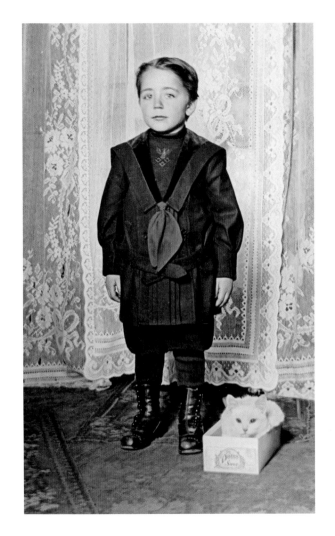
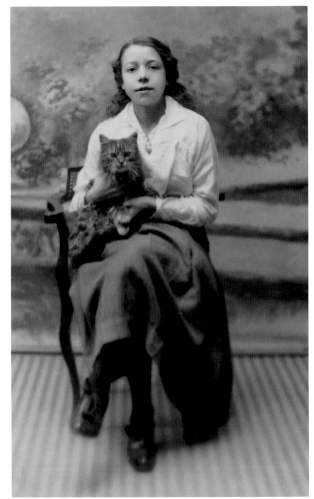

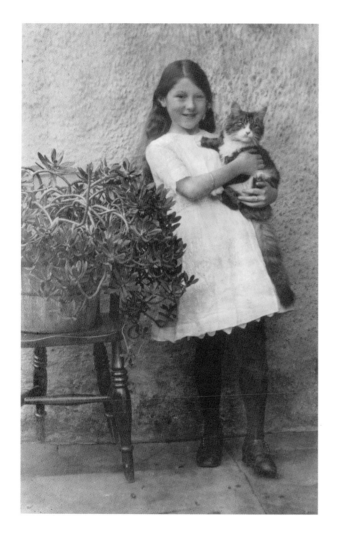

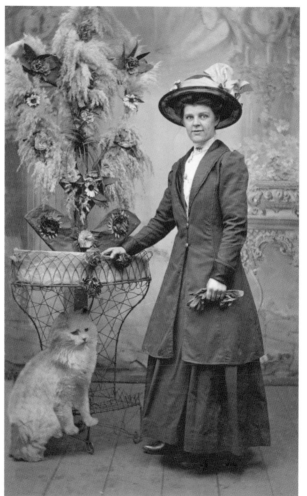

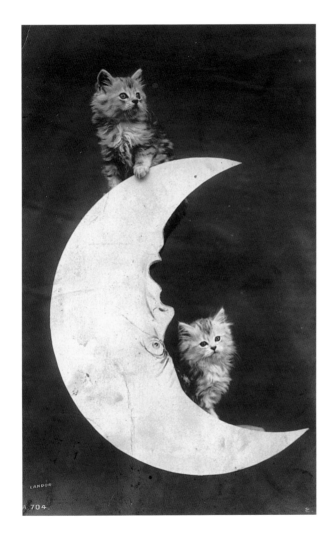

LANDOR

A 704.

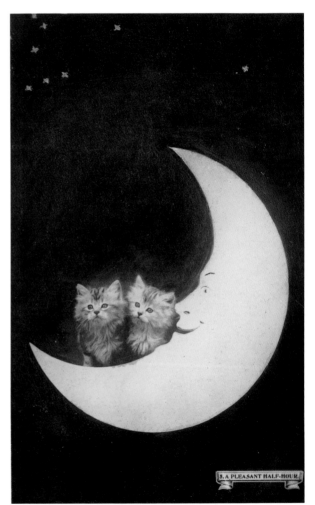

5. A PLEASANT HALF-HOUR.

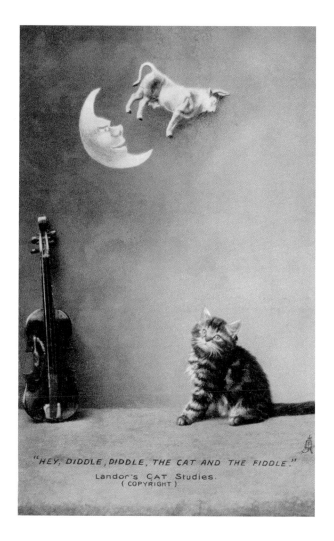

"HEY, DIDDLE, DIDDLE, THE CAT AND THE FIDDLE."
Landor's CAT Studies.
(COPYRIGHT)

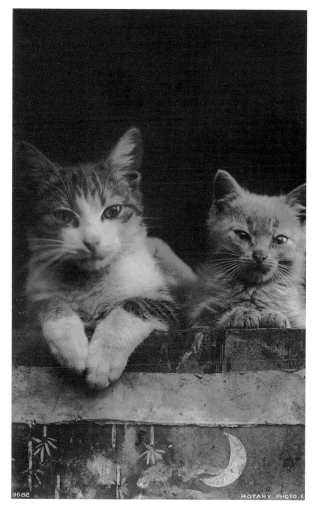

ROTARY PHOTO. E

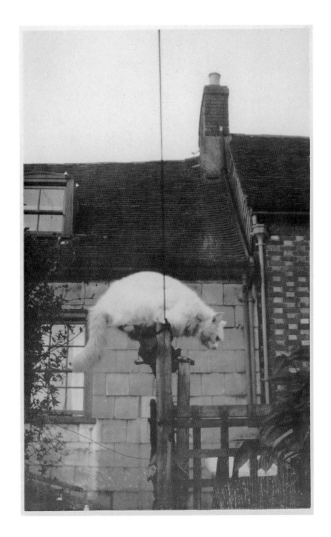 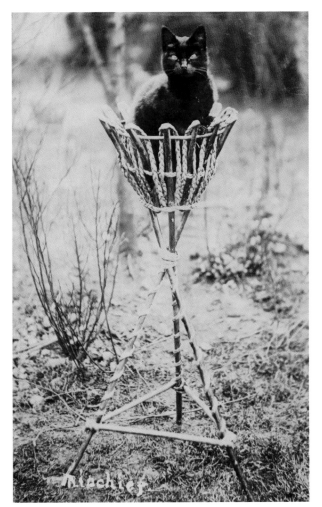

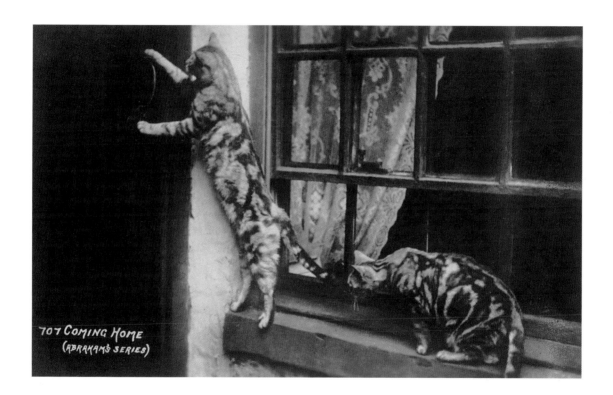

707 Coming Home
(Abrahams Series)

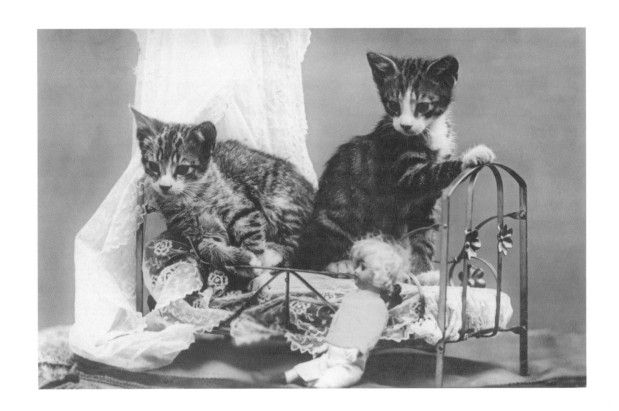

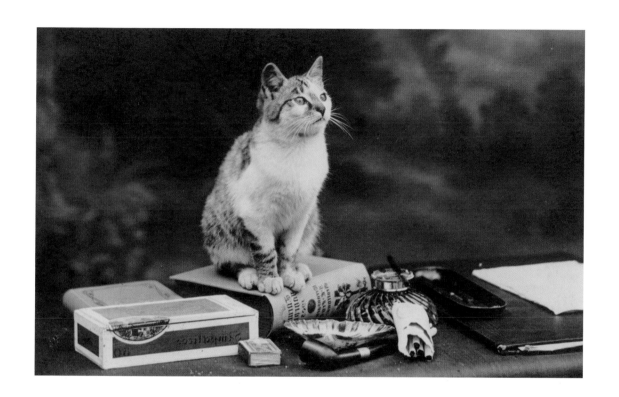

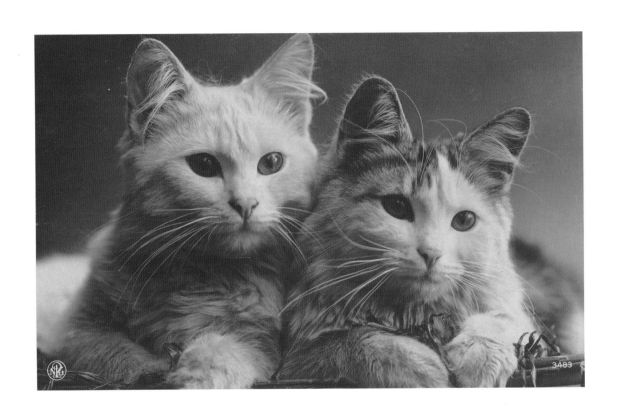

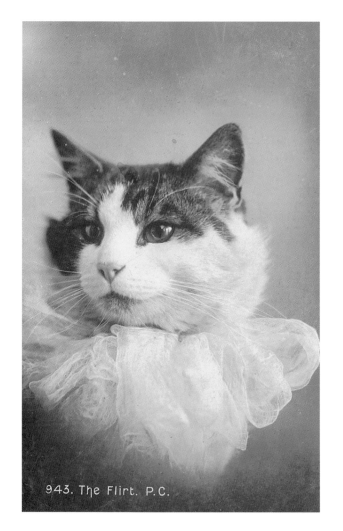

943. The Flirt. P.C.

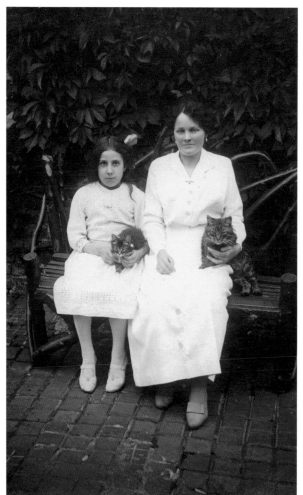

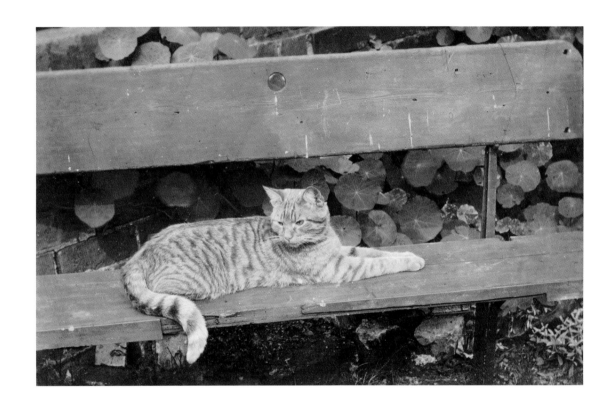

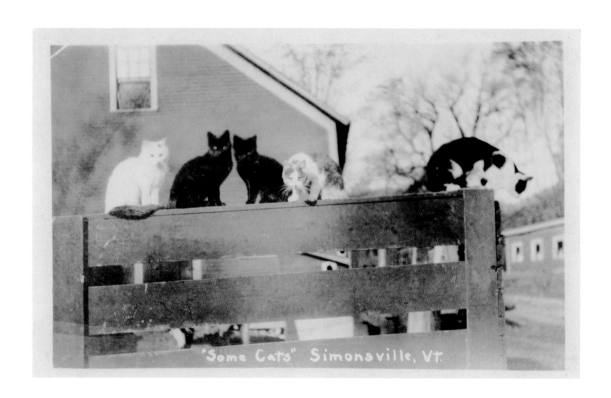

"Some Cats" Simonsville, Vt.

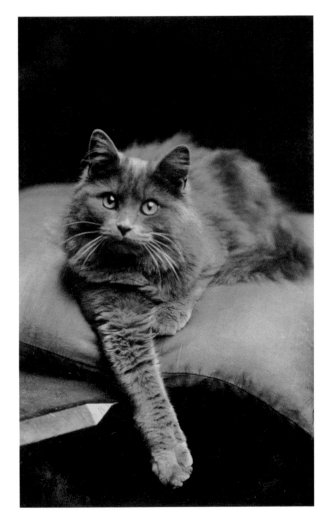

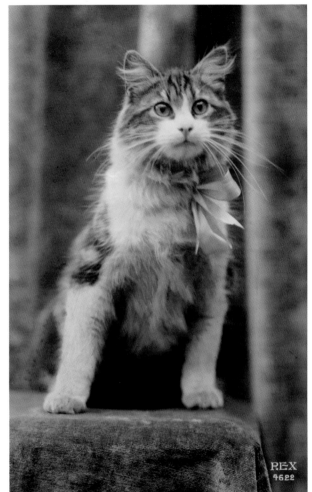

116

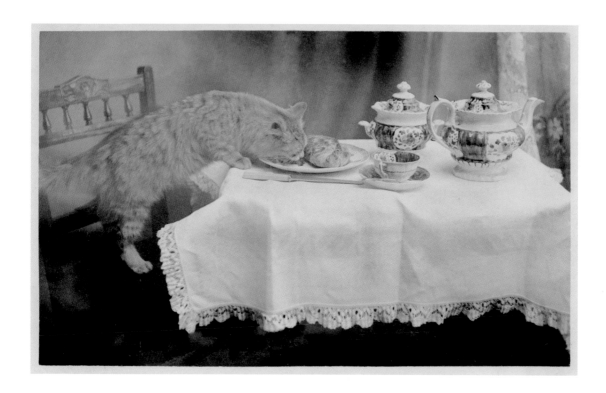

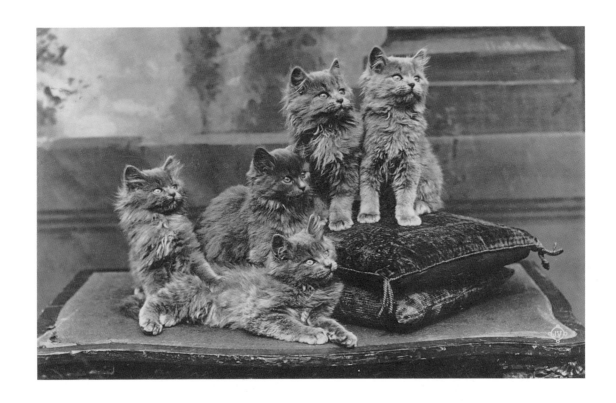

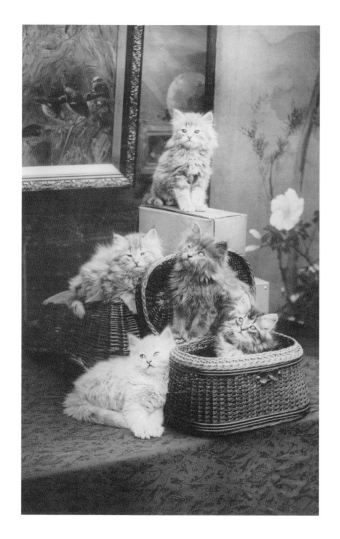

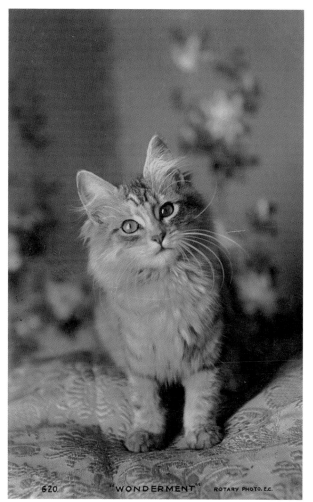

620. "WONDERMENT" ROTARY PHOTO. E.C.

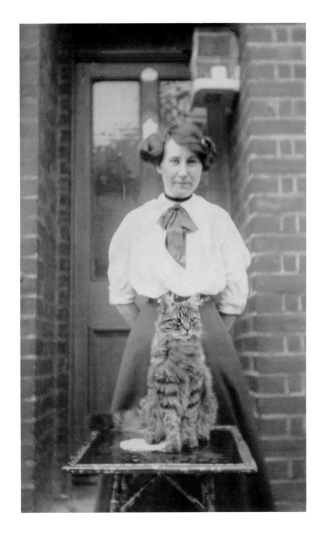

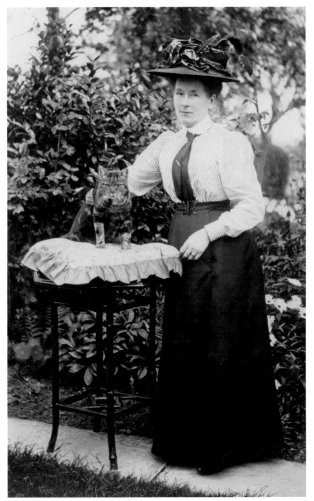

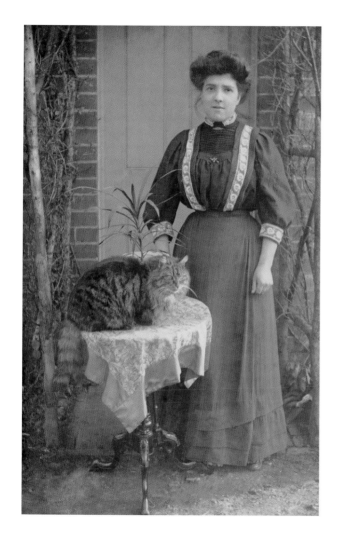
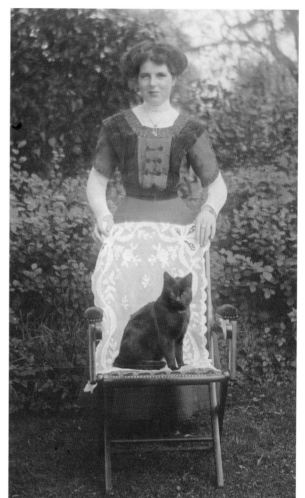

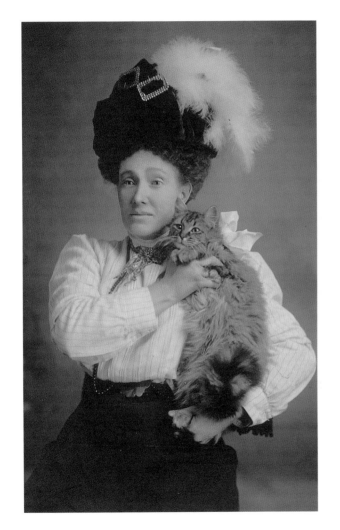
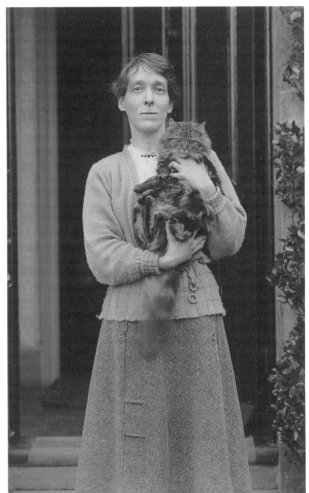

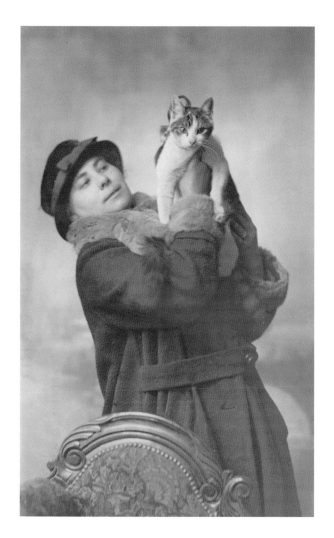

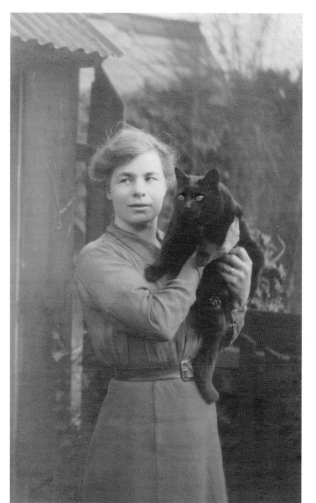

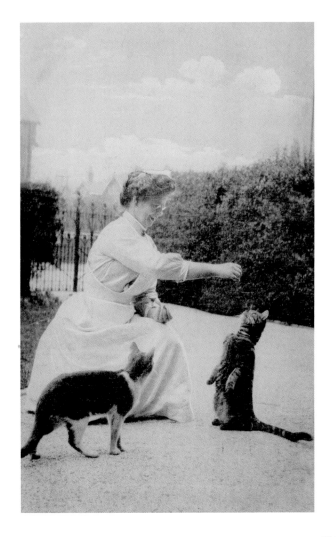

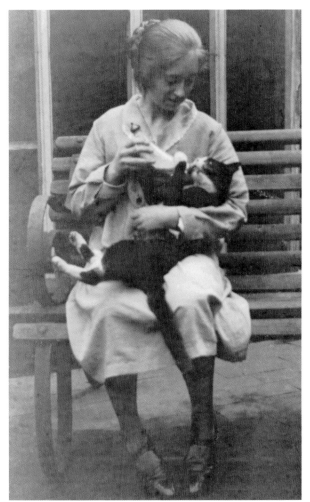

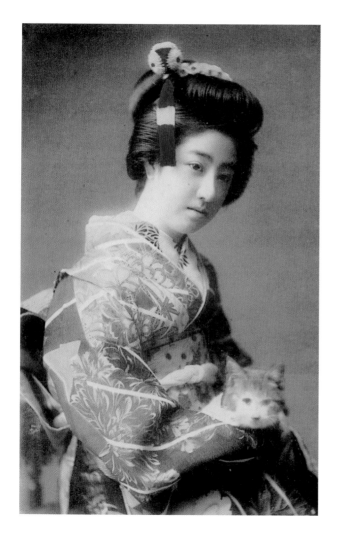
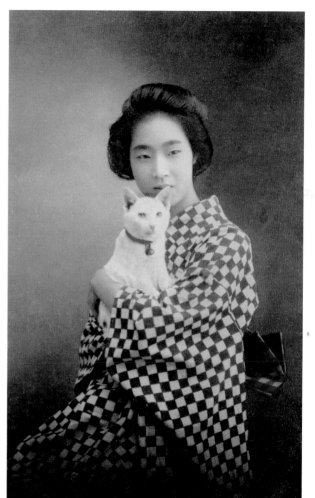

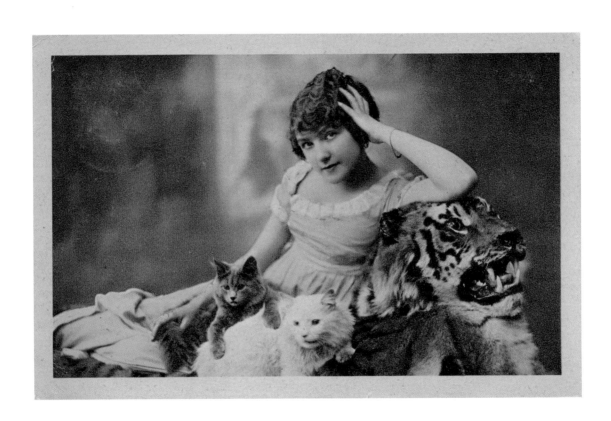

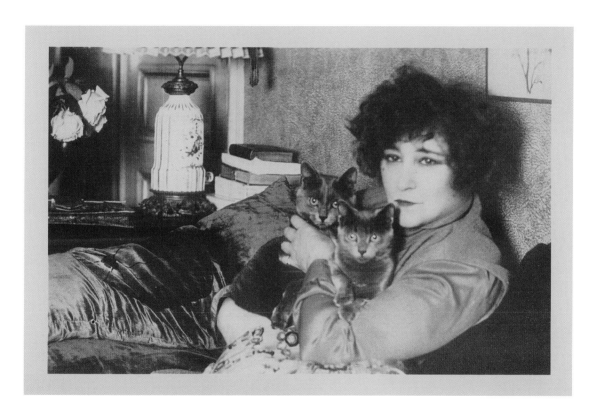

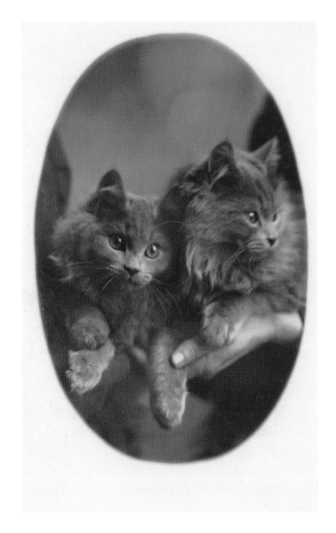

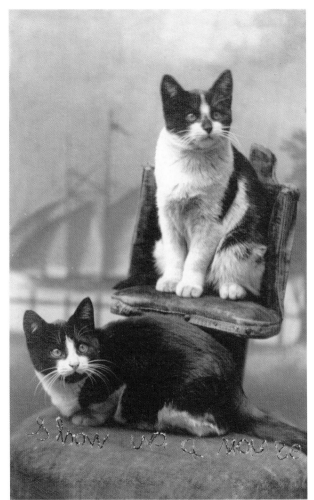

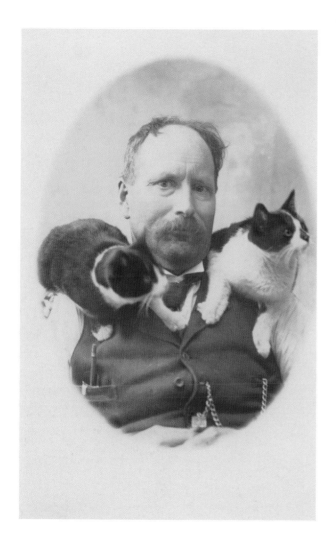
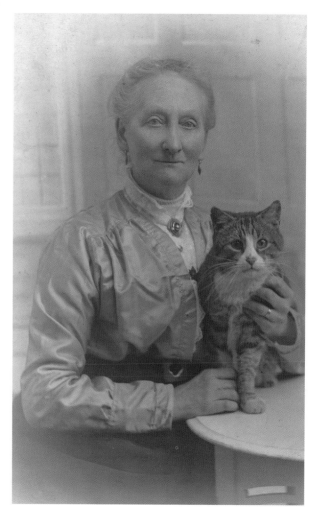

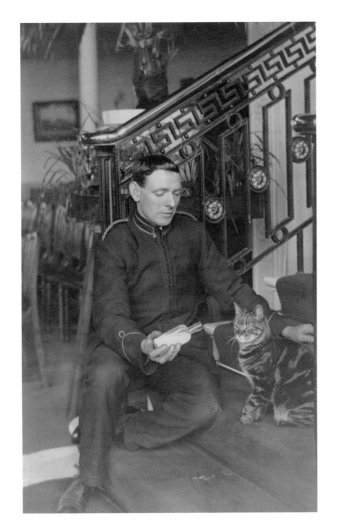

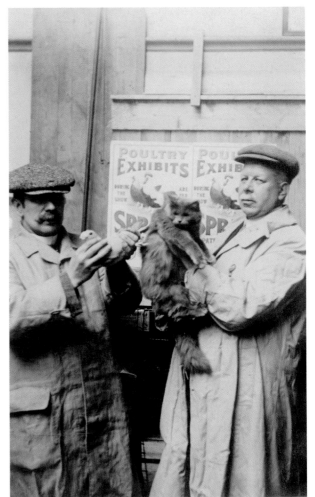

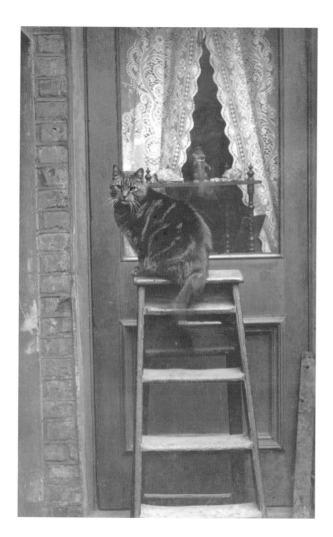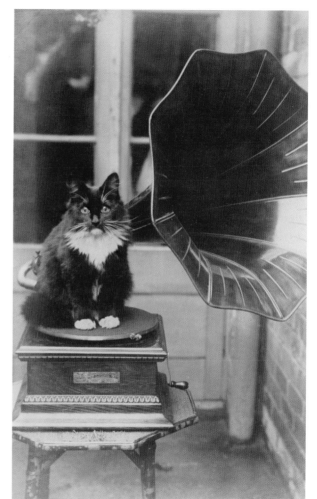

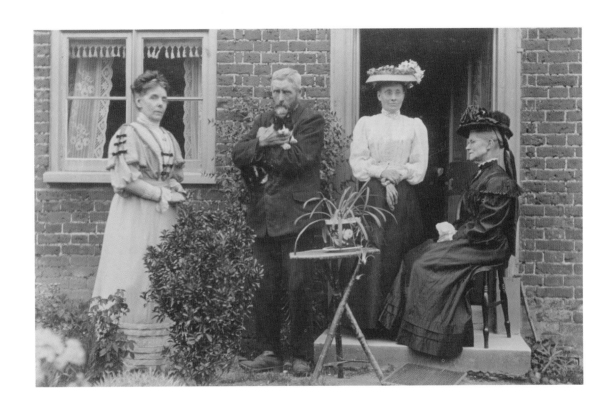

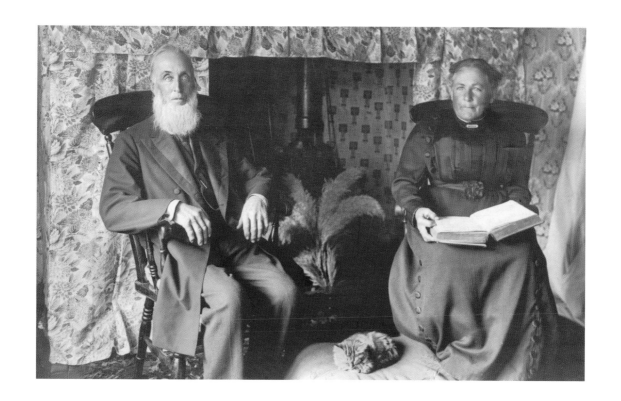

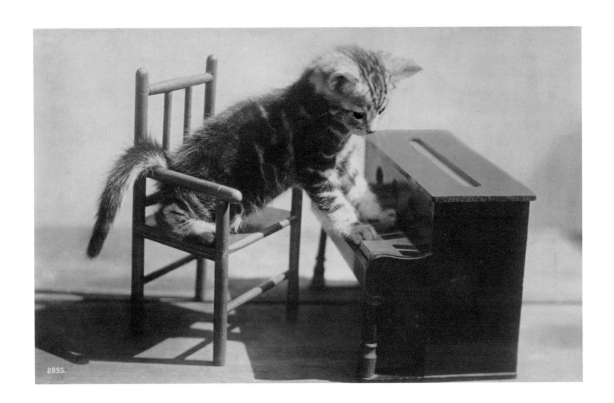

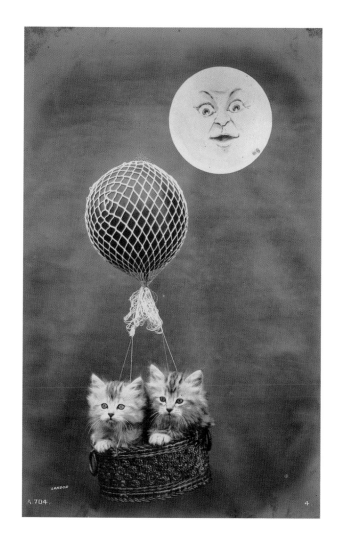

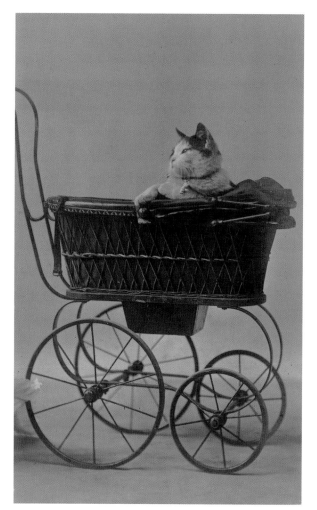

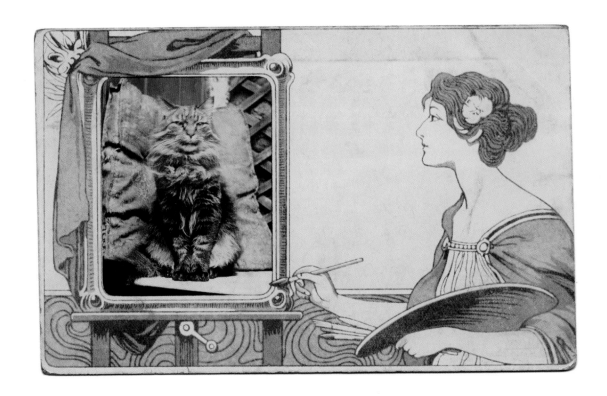

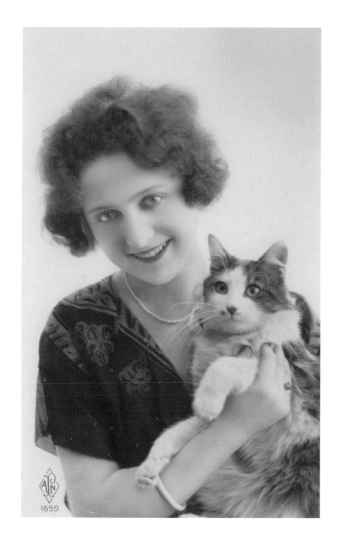

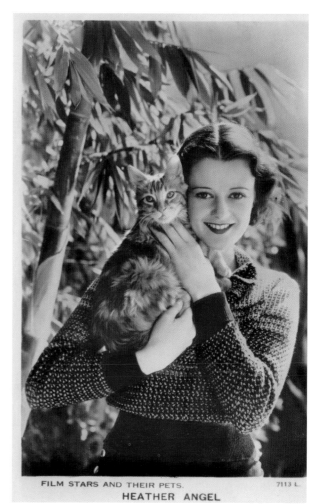

FILM STARS AND THEIR PETS.

7113 L.

HEATHER ANGEL

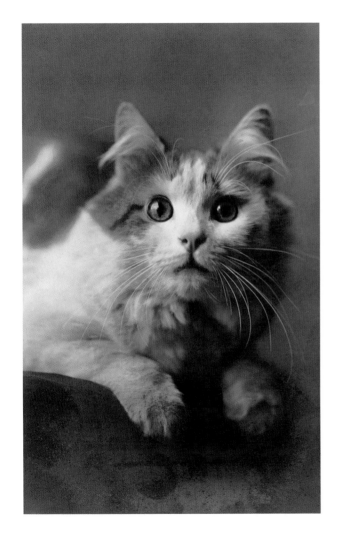

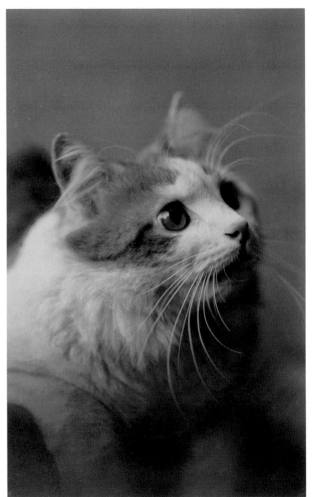

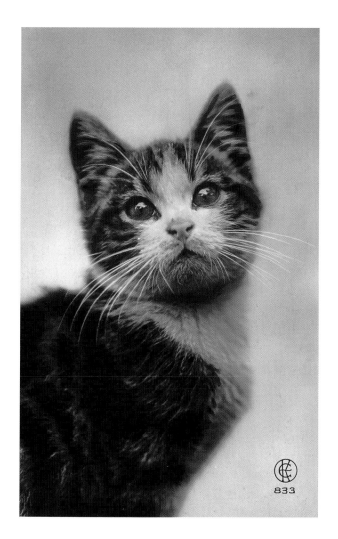

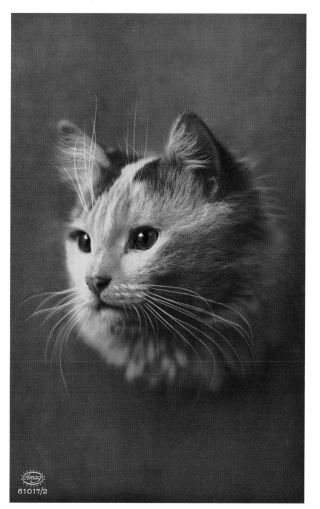

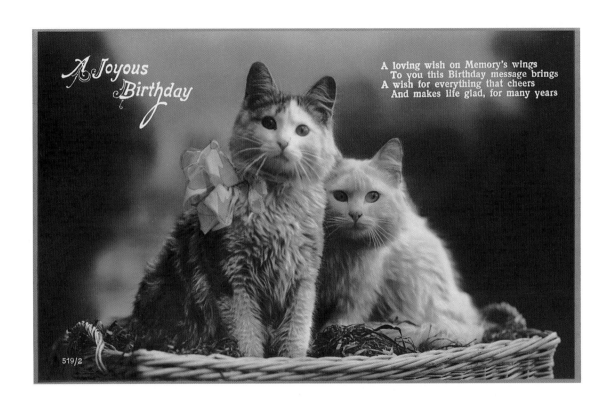

A Joyous Birthday

A loving wish on Memory's wings
To you this Birthday message brings
A wish for everything that cheers
And makes life glad, for many years

519/2

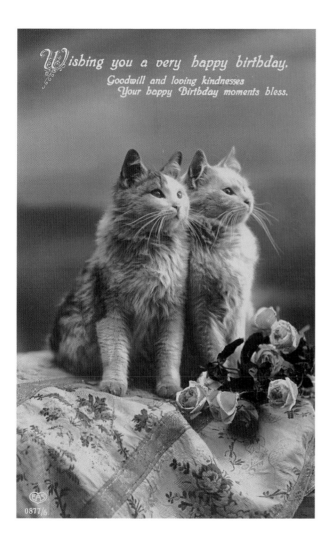

Wishing you a very happy birthday.

Goodwill and loving kindnesses
Your happy Birthday moments bless.

0877/6

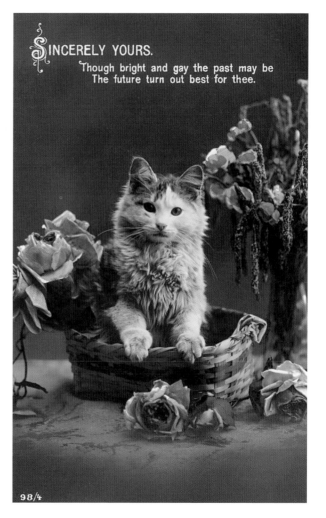

SINCERELY YOURS.

Though bright and gay the past may be
The future turn out best for thee.

98/4

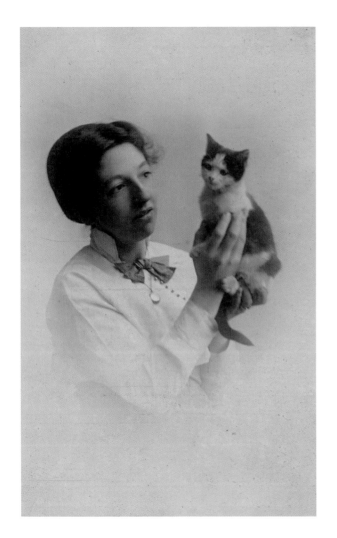

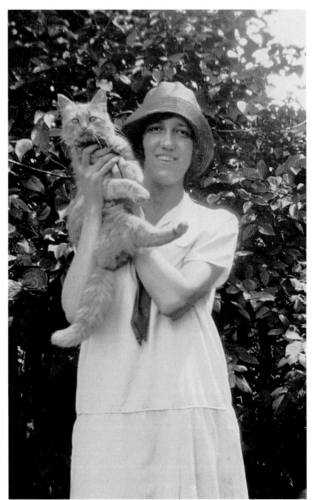

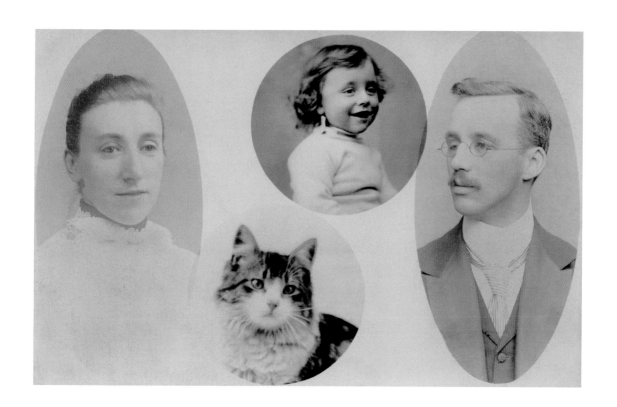

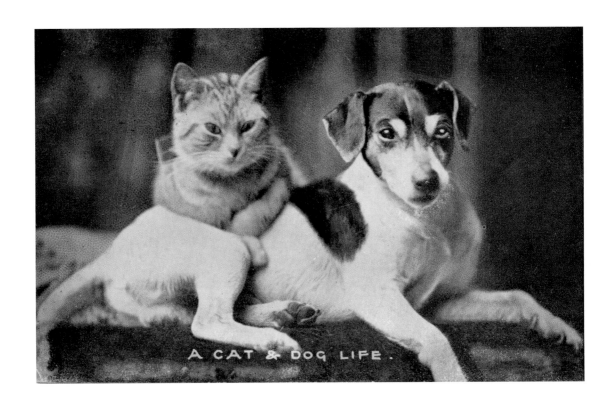

A CAT & DOG LIFE.

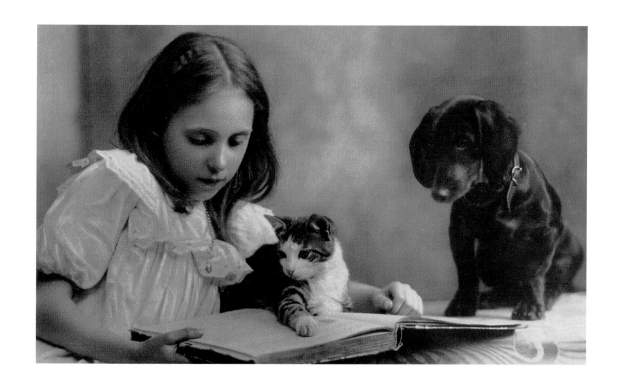

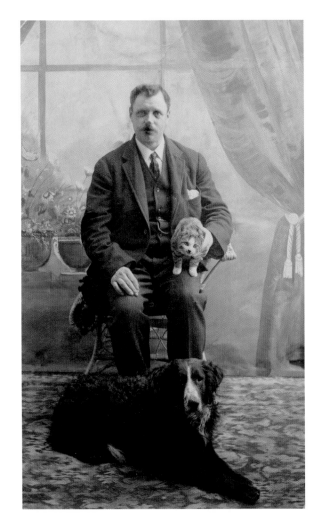

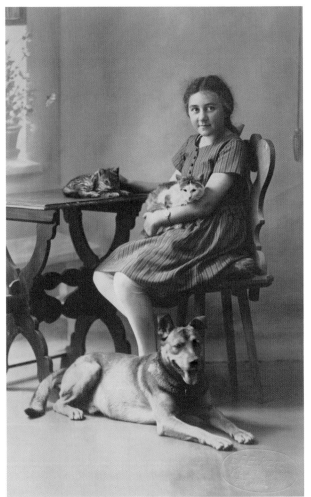

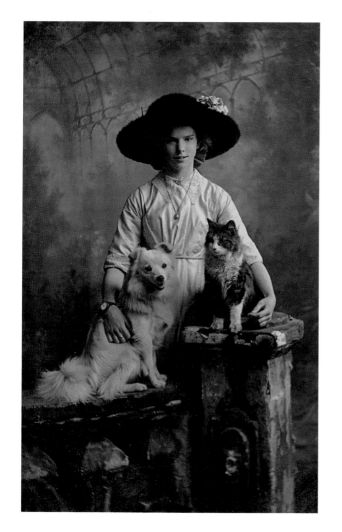

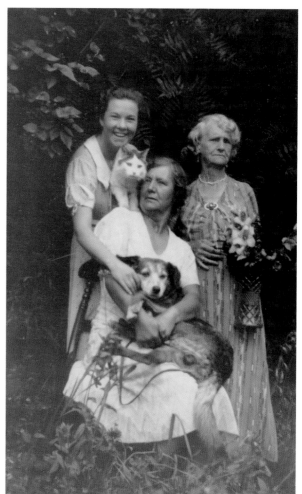

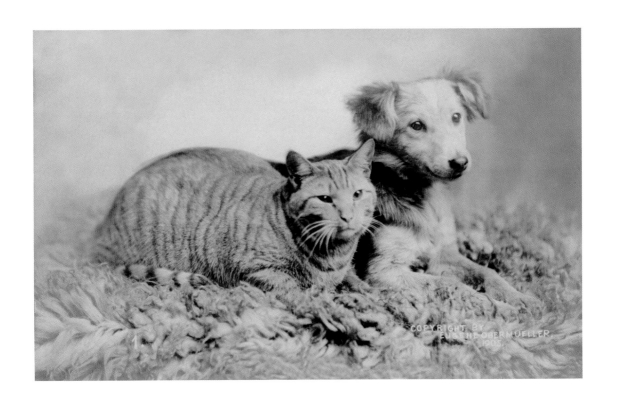

148

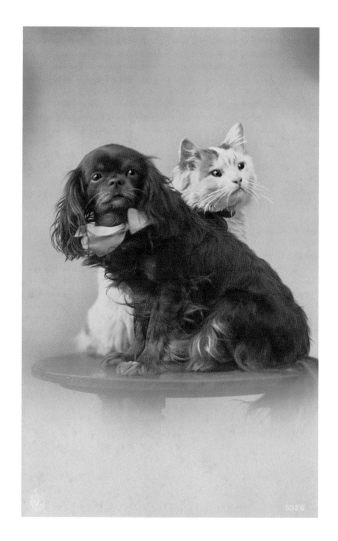

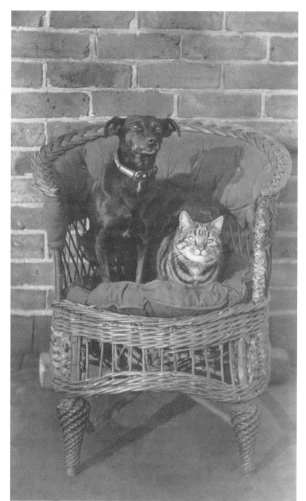

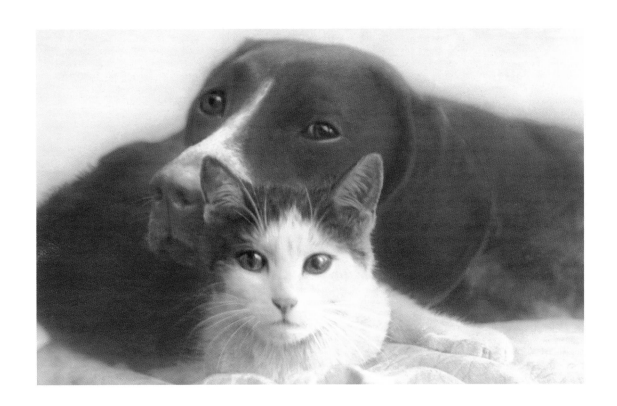

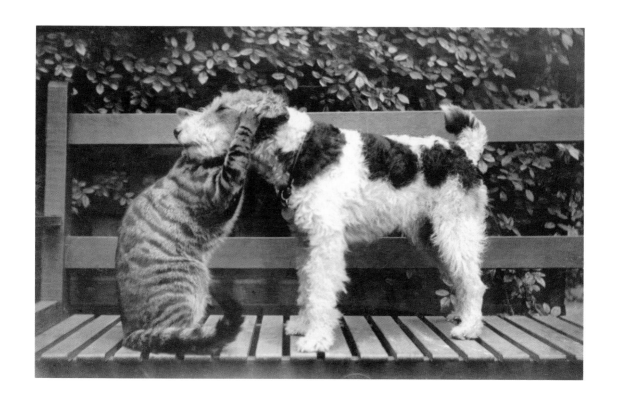

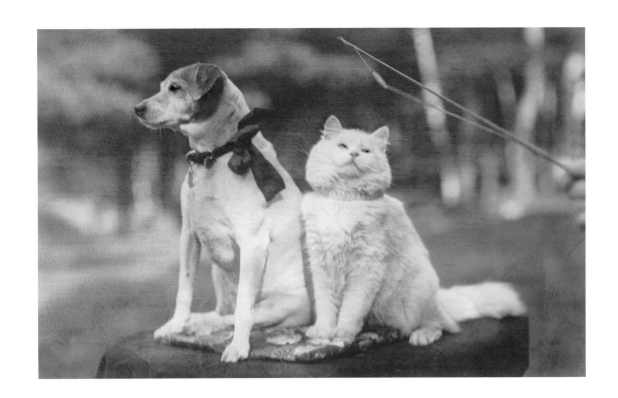

Thank you to Liz Calder and Bloomsbury, to Tony Hall, Alice Wood, Bill Osborne,
James Gardiner, Alan Irvine, Bill Hurrell, Patrick Wildgust, and Bill Main,
to all those who have so generously given us postcards to add to our collections,
and to the dealers and collectors who have helped us in our search.

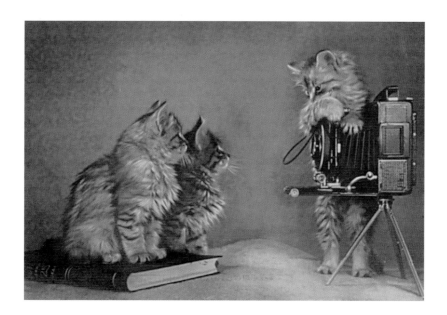

CREDITS AND NOTES

Every attempt has been made to give credit where credit is due. Many private cards, however, and even some that are commercial in style, give no details of source, whether it be publisher, studio or photographer. Where no information is given below, the card is in this sense anonymous. Any copyright information made known to the publishers will be acknowledged in future editions of the book.

2.	*Raphael Tuck & Sons, Art Postcard. Series 864, Landor's cat studies.*
6L.	*Monogram: R.*
11.	*Raphael Tuck & Sons', Real Photograph Postcard.*
12L.	*L. Neurhöfer, Münsingen.*
12R.	*E.E. Flack, Alexandria Bay, N.Y.*
16L.	*Monogram: BNX.*
16R.	*Regina.*
17L. & R.	*The Carlton Publishing Co., London E.C.*
18L.	*Monogram: PHR.*
18R.	*'Does Anybody Want a Cat?' Bamforth Postcard Collection, Leeds, LS10 1JP.*
19L.	*Marque Étoile, 2 rue d'Amsterdam, Paris.*
19R.	*'Good Morning'. Bamforth Postcard Collection, Leeds, LS10 1JP.*
20L.	*'Will No One Play With Me?' Rotary Photographic Series.*
20R.	*The Rotograph Co., N.Y. City.*
21L.	*The Rotograph Co., N.Y. City.*
21R.	*Reutlinger, Paris.*
22.	*Coloured Bromide Studies Series 6830.*
24.	*Monogram: PH.*
25.	*Valentine's X.L. Series. Real Photo Cards.*
27L.	*Courrier, Paris.*
27R.	*Monogram: PHR.*
28L.	Handwritten note verso: Photograph by Thomas Whitehead.
28R.	*I.M.P. Portrait Co., Earl's Court.*
30.	*Marcuse Day & Co. Ltd, London E.C.*
31.	*Marcuse Day & Co. Ltd, London E.C.*
32L.	*S.J. Harding, Clanfield.*
32R.	*Polo.*
33R.	*S.W. Platter, Photographer, Hanslope, Devon.*
34R.	*Lessey Beard FRPS. The Clevedon Studio.*
36L.	*Photographer unknown.* Handwritten note verso: Taken Jan 31/12 Douglas Alaska.
39L.	Photo by Cleeves, Bognor Regis.
42L. & R.	*Monogram: GL Co/PRA.*
43.	*Monogram: GL Co/PRA.*
44L.	*Bamforth Postcard Collection, Leeds, LS10 1JP.*
44R.	*Rotary Photographic Series.*
45L.	*Rotary Photo, London E.C./ Malcolm Arbuthnot.*
45R.	*Charles Voisey, London.*
47.	*Monogram: PL, Paris.*
48.	*Lévy Fils & Cie, Paris. Mésange.*
49L.	*Monogram: AN [or HN?], Paris.*
49R.	*Mésange.*
50.	*The Rapid Photo Printing Co. Ltd, London, E.C.*
51L.	*Ettlinger's Handcoloured Brown Toned Art Studies.*

52R.	Millar & Lang, Ltd. Art Publishers, Glasgow and London.
53.	Le bon éditeur.
54L.	Monogram: RTB.
54R.	PC, Paris.
55.	'An Early Morning Call'. The Rapid Photo Printing Co. Ltd, London, E.C. Bunnett.
56L.	The Heinemann Studio, Preston, Iowa.
56R.	Hermann Tietz, München.
57L.	J. Baxter, Castleford.
58L.	'What lovely fur, / but I prefer / sweet lips like this. / Let's love & kiss.' Dix 1239/2 Visé, Paris.
58R.	Mésange. Lévy Fils & Cie, Paris.
59L.	Marque Étoile, 2 rue d'Amsterdam, Paris. V B C série.
59R	Lepogravure. Monogram: LEP.
60L.	The Alpha Postcard.
60R.	'Our Pet'. The London View Co. Ltd.
61L.	'The bird fancier'. Croissant, Paris.
61R.	EFA. Animal Studies. Photo E. Hawthorn.
62L.	Monogram: GLO.
62R.	'Miss Gabrielle Ray'. Rotary Photographic Series, Foulsham & Banfield.
63L.	'Miss Marie Studholme'. Rotary Photographic Series, W. & D. Downey. London S.W.
63R.	The Carlton Publishing Co., London E.C.
64L.	Aristophot Co. Ltd, London W.C.
64R.	Judges' Ltd, Hastings.
65L.	The London View Co. Ltd.
66R.	'Gained Any Since?' Rotary Photographic Series.

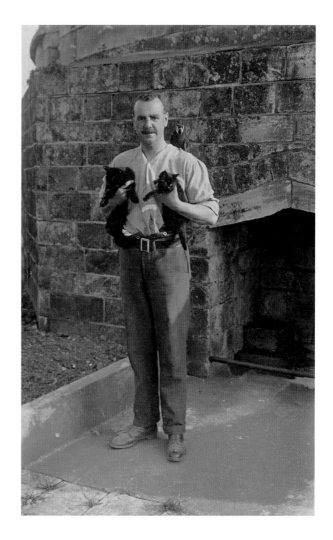

67.	W.E. Mack, London N.W.3.		West Hamilton, Canada.
72.	DIC Photo. 173 Elizabeth St, Hobart.	106L.	Rotary Photographic Series, Landor.
75L.	Stickybacks, 35 Biggin St, Dover, etc.	106R.	Boots Cash Chemist. Real Photograph Series.
79R.	A. & G. Taylor's Orthochrome Series.	107L.	Raphael Tuck & Sons. Photochrome PC Series.
	70 & 78 Queen Victoria St, London E.C.		Cat Studies.
80L. & R.	J. Easton, Clifton Baths, Margate.	107R.	'Shall We Come?' Rotary Photographic Series.
81.	Miss M. Kirton, Harris Promenade,	109.	Abraham's, photograph by
	Douglas. I.O.M.		G.P. Abraham Ltd, Keswick.
84.	'Now Who May You Be?'	111.	Lohmann, Asnières.
	Rotary Photographic Series, Landor.	112.	Monogram: NGP.
85L.	Acourrier, Paris.		Published by M.T. Sheahan, Boston.
85R.	The Carlton Publishing Co., London E.C.	116.	'A Thief in the House No 12'. S. Dalby-Smith's
86.	Rotary Photo E.C.		Photo. St. Blazey, Cornwall.
87L.	M.T. Sheahan Publisher, Boston, Mass.	117L.	'Blue Persian II'. J. J. Samuels, Post Card Depôts,
87R.	Rotary Photographic Series.	150	Strand & 97a Regent St.
88L.	The Rapid Photo Printing Co. Ltd, London. E.C.	117R.	Rex.
88R.	Valentine's Series.	118.	Monogram: JV.
89.	The Rapid Photo Printing Co. Ltd, London. E.C.	119L.	Monogram: JV.
90.	The Carlton Printing Co., London E.C.	119R.	Rotary Photographic Series.
91.	Kiss.	120L.	Thatcher & Son, Photographers, Tadley,
92.	'Maybe It's a Ghost'. Rotary Photographic Series.		Basingstoke.
93.	J. Beagles & Co. Ltd, E.C.	124L.	The Scientific Press Ltd, London.
94.	Raphael Tuck & Sons, Rapholette Glosso.	129L.	Annie R. Gibb, Silloth.
	'In Kittendom' series.	130L.	G.E. Houghton Photo, Broadstairs.
95.	E.A. Schwerdtfeger & Co., London E.C.	134.	The Philco Publishing Co., Holborn Place,
96L.	Rotary Photo, London, E.C.		London, W.C.
96R.	Wildt & Kray Ltd, London, E.C.1.	135L.	Rotary Photo, London E.C.
97L.	Monogram: PFB.	135R.	Hood, Moffat & Lockerbie.
98.	Martin Rommel & Co., Hofkunstanstalt, Stuttgart.	137L.	Monogram: ANP.
103.	A.H. Hardwick, Photographer,	137R.	Valentine.

This of course is primarily a book for those interested in cats. We ought therefore to warn the more rigorous among postcard purists that some images have been cropped or otherwise enhanced to show the featured cats to their best advantage. The occasional mawkish rhyme has been removed as well as the usual creases, spots and stains. While the majority of illustrations show complete cards, our title *Postcard Cats* (as opposed to *Cat Postcards*) would seem to imply a certain licence to give the cats priority.

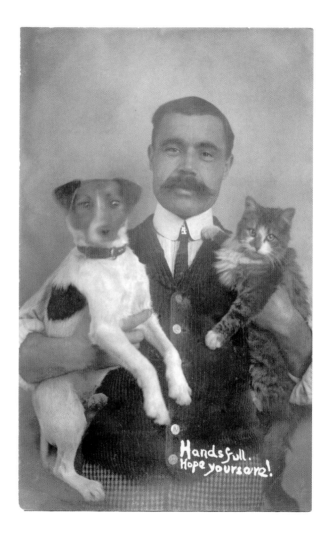

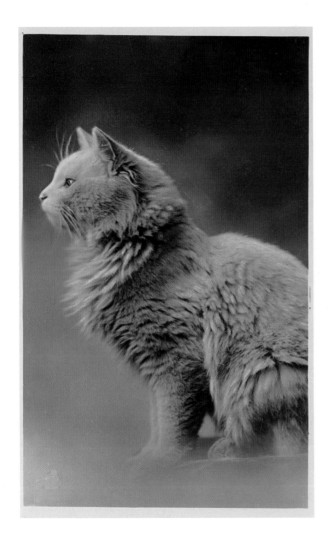

Although there are a few shops selling postcards, most dealing is done in the numerous postcard fairs that take place, both in Britain and the United States, in various venues at weekends throughout the year. In continental Europe, especially in France, street markets are also popular places to buy. In recent years, of course, the internet has become an ever more lively forum for buying and selling, but for getting to know the field there is no substitute for actually handling the cards and talking to the dealers. Most of the cards in this book have been found by such means. Those interested particularly in cards featuring cats will find that the majority of dealers at fairs have a specially designated section to comb through, but it is always worthwhile to seach in miscellaneous boxes of cheaper cards. In the UK the best source of information is the excellent *Picture Postcard Monthly* published by Reflections, 15 Debdale Lane, Keyworth, Nottingham NG12 5HT, whose *Picture Postcard Annual* lists all the fairs for the year and gives a useful guide to postcard-hunting in other countries.

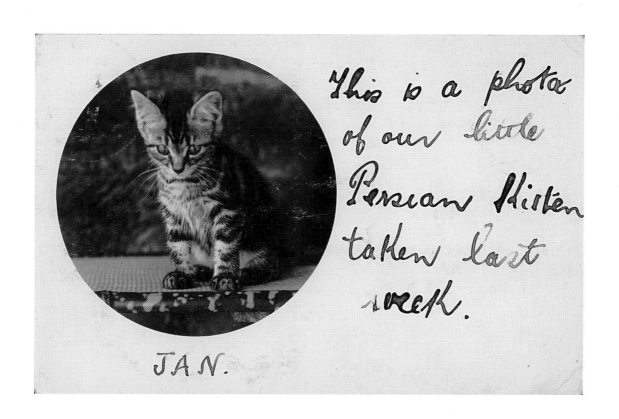

This is a photo
of our little
Persian kitten
taken last
week.

JAN.

Also by LIBBY HALL

Prince and Other Dogs 1850–1940 London and New York, Bloomsbury, 2000
Prince and Other Dogs II London and New York, Bloomsbury, 2002
Postcard Dogs London and New York, Bloomsbury, 2004

Also by TOM PHILLIPS

The Postcard Century London and New York, Thames & Hudson, 2000
We are the People London, National Portrait Gallery, 2004

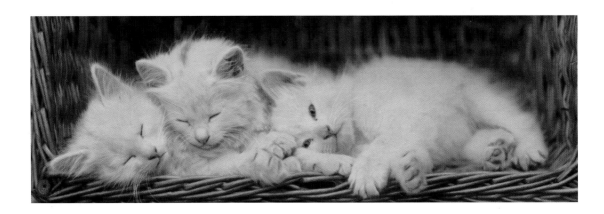